SOCIAL CHANGE, PUBLIC POLICY, AND COMMUNITY COLLABORATIONS

Training Human Development Professionals For the Twenty-First Century

OUTREACH SCHOLARSHIP

Editor:

Richard M. Lerner
Tufts University
Medford, Massachusetts, U.S.A.

SOCIAL CHANGE, PUBLIC POLICY, AND COMMUNITY COLLABORATIONS
Training Human Development Professionals For the Twenty-First Century

edited by

Penny A. Ralston
Florida State University U.S.A.

Richard M. Lerner
Tufts University U.S.A.

Ann K. Mullis
Florida State University U.S.A.

Coby B. Simerly
Florida State University U.S.A.

John P. Murray
Kansas State University U.S.A .

KLUWER ACADEMIC PUBLISHERS
Boston / Dordrecht / London

Distributors for North, Central and South America:
Kluwer Academic Publishers
101 Philip Drive
Assinippi Park
Norwell, Massachusetts 02061 USA
Telephone (781) 871-6600
Fax (781) 871-6528
E-Mail <kluwer@wkap.com>

Distributors for all other countries:
Kluwer Academic Publishers Group
Distribution Centre
Post Office Box 322
3300 AH Dordrecht, THE NETHERLANDS
Telephone 31 78 6392 392
Fax 31 78 6546 474
E-Mail <services@wkap.nl>

 Electronic Services <http://www.wkap.nl>

Library of Congress Cataloging-in-Publication Data

Social change, public policy, and community collaborations: training human
development professionals for the twenty-first century / edited by Penny A. Ralston...[et al.].
    p. cm. -- (Outreach scholarship; 3)
    Includes biobliographical references and index.
    ISBN 0-7923-8659-0 (alk. paper)
    1. Human services--Study and teaching (Higher)-- Congresses. 2. Human services
personnel--Training of--Congresses. 3. Social policy--Study and teaching
(Higher)--Congresses. 4.Community and college--Congresses. I.Ralston, Penny A. II.
Series.

HV11 .S58544 1999
361'.0071'173--dc21
                                                                99-046690

Printed on acid-free paper.   Printed in the United States of America

Contents

SECTION I   Introduction: A View of the Issues

SECTION II   Dimensions of Training and Community Collaboration

List of Figures

List of Contributors

Barbara Ash, Coordinator of Communications, Office of the Vice President for Research, Florida State University

W. J. Blechman, Lawton & Rhea Chiles Center for Healthy Mothers & Babies

Norma Burgess, Chair, Child and Family Studies, College for Human Development, Syracuse University

The Honorable Lawton Chiles, Governor of Florida, 1991-1998

Karen E. Craig, Dean, College of Human Resources and Family Sciences, University of Nebraska-Lincoln

Martha Farrell Erickson, Director, Children, Youth and Family Consortium, University of Minnesota

Golden Jackson, Assistant Professor, Consumer and Textile Sciences, College of Human Ecology, Ohio State University

Joan M. Laughlin, Associate Dean, Research and Graduate Studies, College of Human Resources and Family Sciences, University of Nebraska

Richard M. Lerner, Bergstrom Chair in Applied Developmental Science, Eliot-Pearson Department of Child Development, Tufts University

Jack Levine, Executive Director, Center for Florida's Children

Connie Ley, Professor, Department of Family and Consumer Sciences, Illinois State University

Charles McClintock, Professor and Associate Dean, College of Human Ecology, Cornell University

Julia Miller, Dean, College of Human Ecology, Michigan State University

Ann K. Mullis, Associate Professor, Department of Family and Child Sciences, College of Human Sciences, Florida State University

John P. Murray, Professor and Interim Associate Vice Provost for Research, Kansas State University

Clara Pratt, Professor and Knudson Endowed Chair in Family Policy, Family Studies Center, Oregon State University

Penny A. Ralston, Professor and Dean, College of Human Sciences, Florida State University

x

Social Change, Public Policy, and Community Collaborations: Training
Human Development Professionals for the Twenty-First Century

Catherine J. Ross, Associate Professor of Law, George Washington University

Ulrike Schuermann, Executive Director, The Australian Youth Foundation, Inc.

Lonnie R. Sherrod, Executive Vice President, William T. Grant Foundation

Coby S. Simerly, former Associate Professor and Associate Dean for Outreach, College of Human Sciences, Florida State University

Denise Skinner, Professor, Department of Human Development, Family Living and Community Educational Services, College of Human Development, University of Wisconsin-Stout

Bea Smith, Dean, College of Human Environmental Sciences, University of Missouri-Columbia

James C. Votruba, President, Northern Kentucky University

Richard A. Weinberg, Birkmaier Professor of Educational Leadership, Professor of Child Psychology, Director of the Institute of Child Development, University of Minnesota

Brian L. Wilcox, Professor of Psychology, Director, Center on Children, Families and the Law, University of Nebraska-Lincoln

Foreword[1]
Lawton Chiles
Governor of Florida, 1991-1998

Social Change, Public Policy and Community Collaborations: Training Human Development Professionals for the Twenty-First Century is more than the name of the Third National Applied Developmental Science Conference; it is more than the name of a book prepared from the proceedings of this conference. It describes one of the largest and most complex challenges facing state government, higher education and communities in the coming decade.

The answer to this challenge will not be found in a college or program in our higher education institution nor in laws conceived and written in state capitals. The answers to this challenge are to be found at the place where academia, public policy, and communities meet.

The problems and issues that are facing our children and families will require that all the players work together to develop community-driven programs, designed and evaluated using current research and staffed by highly trained professionals. It will be critical that academia, policy makers, legislators, and community members work together to ensure that the programs we design work. We must ensure that research is being conducted so that programs that work better are continued and programs that don't are stopped.

The training provided to the professionals in these programs will look very different from the traditional training of decades past. The training will cross over "college" lines more than ever before. The training will include a greater emphasis on public policy and its formation, be more competency-based and will be strongly rooted in community experiences. These highly trained professionals will then have access to a system of professional compensation that supports retention and continued training.

No governor, state legislator, university administrator or professor alone has all the answers to solving the problems communities face. We must look to our communities, and working together with them, provide the information and resources they need to meet the challenges they face.

Almost daily, we are learning more and more about how children develop, the role of parents in this development, and the interventions and services that support healthy development. This information must be used by higher education, government leaders and community members to inform our activities. The information must be used to develop and sustain programs that train professionals who will be providing support to our families; to help parents as they undertake the hardest job anyone can imagine—raising a child.

We must ensure that we have professionals trained to address the needs of the young parent receiving government assistance who is being required to return to work when the child is three months old.

We must ensure that we have professionals trained to protect our children from abuse and neglect. We ask these professionals to make tough decisions every day. We must commit to ensuring that these professionals in whom we vest so much responsibility have the training and resources to do the job well.

xii

Social Change, Public Policy, and Community Collaborations: Training
Human Development Professionals for the Twenty-First Century

We must invest in professionals who will ensure that our children are born healthy, raised healthy and stay healthy; who will teach our children in increasingly complex school settings; and who will care for our youngest and most vulnerable citizens in our child care centers. In fact, we must be prepared to invest in training and education for roles we have not even thought of yet.

It is a huge responsibility that is being placed on all of us. But we must shoulder this responsibility because the future of our children, our families and our communities will depend on it.

NOTE

1. Lawton Chiles died unexpectedly on December 12, 1998. The foreword to this book was one of his last written documents.

Preface

The children of our nation, and the families and communities that seek to nurture their healthy development, face a set of challenges that are at historically troublesome levels. Whether we focus on the striking co-occurrence of risk behaviors, or the alarming rates of youth poverty—now involving a fifth of our nation's children and adolescents—or on the continuing gender, racial, and ethnic inequities in our society, it is clear that our communities need to have greater access to existing and effective programs serving family and youth (see, for example, Dryfoos, 1998; Hamburg, 1992; Schorr, 1997). Moreover, we need to develop policies and practices that sustain the existing programs and support the development of new innovative programs (Lerner, 1995; Lerner & Galambos, 1998).

The goal of this book is to provide a discussion of the ways in which universities, communities, and policy makers can create partnerships to foster community-university collaborations that promote the positive development of youth and families. Second, the book seeks to sustain these efforts through educating a new cadre of professionals who can further build effective community-based programs and policies. Based on the vision of scholarship involved in the human sciences, and the work being pursued in the disciplines involved in applied developmental science, the contributors to this volume propose ideas about creating caring communities through broad, multi-disciplinary, multi-professional, multi-institutional, and citizen-led collaborations. We believe universities can play a central role in initiating these collaborations and in the provision of training for community leaders who are dedicated to building the capacity of citizens to promote positive development of children and families in our nation's diverse communities.

This volume is derived from presentations and discussions among participants in the Third National Conference on Applied Developmental Science (ADS), held at Florida State University in March, 1997. The conference, "Social change, public policy, and community collaboration: Training human development professionals for the twenty-first century," was co-sponsored by the American Association of Family and Consumer Sciences Higher Education Unit (AAFCS-HEU), the Association of Administrators of Human Sciences (AAHS), the National Task Force on Applied Developmental Science, and the Family Institute in the College of Human Sciences at Florida State University, along with other academic units at the university. The present volume expands on the conference theme by providing scholarship aimed at changing the character of graduate and undergraduate education in human development-related disciplines pertinent to public policy engagement. To undergird and sustain this reorientation in education, we include ideas for transforming the character of higher education and its administration in the direction of promoting co-learning and collaboration between universities and the communities they serve.

We hope that the integration of ideas about undergraduate and graduate education, about university administrative and scholarly transformations that are aimed at involving higher education more collaboratively in the lives of children and families, and about the engagement of public policy constitute a useful and timely contribution to what has been termed the scholarship of engagement (Boyer,

1990, 1994; Glassick, Taylor-Huber & Smaeroff, 1997) or outreach scholarship (Lerner, 1995). We believe that such scholarship may help our nation's universities move into greater alignment with the issues and aspirations of the American public, as Bok (1990) has urged. As such, universities will make new value-added contributions to the communities within which they are located and, through such service, will enhance civil society in our nation. Indeed, the concept of "adding value" to both the education of students and the communities supporting our universities is an emerging theme among public and private universities across America. For example, Kansas State University recently published a report (Trewyn & Garrett, 1998) documenting a $2.4 billion impact on the State of Kansas as a result of teaching and research that engages public service addressing community needs.

We wish to acknowledge our appreciation of and gratitude to the numerous colleagues who collaborated with us in the development of this book. We owe our greatest debt to the participants and the sponsors of the Third National ADS Conference and to the contributors to this volume. Their intellectual generativity and commitment to use developmental science to promote university-community collaborations and to engage public policy in the service of our nation's youth and families provided unparalleled stimulation and motivation for the editors.

We wish to thank as well Sofia T. Romero, Editor at the Boston College Center for Child, Family, and Community Partnerships, for her skillful editorial guidance and her wise counsel about manuscript development. We are greatly indebted as well to Maggi Vanos-Wilson, Executive Assistant to the Dean of the College of Human Sciences at Florida State University, for coordinating the communications with the contributors to the book and for playing a central role in the final production of the manuscript.

We appreciate also the collaboration of our editors at Kluwer Academic Publishers: Robert Chametzky, Michael Williams, and Scott Delman. Their enthusiasm for this book was a great source of encouragement. We are pleased that the book is part of Kluwer's Outreach Scholarship Series.

We extend our deep gratitude as well to Catherine Ross, Professor of Law at George Washington University, and to James C. Votruba, President of the University of Northern Kentucky, for their generous afterwords to the volume. We deeply appreciate their support of the scholarship pursued by the contributors to this volume and the compelling nature of their respective visions for enhancing community-university collaboration and policy engagement on behalf of youth and families.

In particular, we are grateful to the late Governor Lawton Chiles of Florida, who graciously contributed a foreword to this book. It is fitting that, in what was perhaps his last written pronouncement as governor, he underscored his life-long commitment to children and their families, and, as well, stressed the significance of creating the partnerships among policy makers, universities, and the diverse communities of our nation that are the focus of this book. In marked appreciation of his vision and leadership, we gratefully dedicate this book to him and to the other courageous political leaders whom we are certain he inspired to devote their energies to supporting America's most important group of non-voting citizens: its children.

Penny A. Ralston, *Florida State University*
Richard M. Lerner, *Tufts University*
Ann K. Mullis, *Florida State University*
Coby S. Simerly, *Florida State University*
John P. Murray, *Kansas State University*

REFERENCES

Bok, D. (1990). *Universities and the future of America*. Durham, NC: Duke University Press.

Boyer, E. L. (1990). *Scholarship reconsidered: Priorities of the professoriate*. Princeton, NJ: The Carnegie Foundation for the Advancement of Teaching.

Boyer, E. L. (1994, March 9). Creating the new American college. *The Chronicle of Higher Education*, A48.

Dryfoos, J. G. (1998). *Safe passage: Making it through adolescence in a risky society*. New York: Oxford University Press.

Glassick, C. E., Taylor-Huber, M. & Smaeroff, G. I. (1997). *Scholarship assessed: Evaluation of the professoriate*. San Francisco: Jossey Bass.

Hamburg, D. A. (1992). *Today's children: Creating a future for a generation in crisis*. New York: Time Books.

Lerner, R. M. (1995). *America's youth in crisis: Challenges and options for programs and policies*. Thousand Oaks, CA: Sage.

Lerner, R. M. & Galambos, N. L. (1998). Adolescent development: Challenges and opportunities for research, programs, and policies. In J. T. Spence (Ed.), *Annual Review of Psychology* (Vol. 49, pp. 413-446). Palo Alto, CA: Annual Reviews.

Schorr, L. B. (1997). *Common purpose: Strengthening families and neighborhoods to rebuild America*. New York: Doubleday.

Trewyn, R. W. & Garrett, K. (1998). *Value added: The economic impact of teaching and research at Kansas State University*. Manhattan, KS: Kansas State University.

Training Human Development Professionals in Public Policy and Community Collaboration: A View of the Issues

Richard M. Lerner, *Tufts University*
Penny A. Ralston, *Florida State University*
Ann K. Mullis, *Florida State University*
Coby S. Simerly, *Florida State University*
John P. Murray, *Kansas State University*

America, and the communities that comprise it, face a set of problems of historically unprecedented scope and severity. Issues of economic development, environmental quality, health, and health care delivery challenge the current resources and future viability of our nation. Ultimately, all these problems reduce to issues affecting the lives of people and, most dramatically, the youth and families of our nation (Dryfoos, 1998; Schorr, 1997).

We are living at a time in history when children, adolescents, and families in the United States and around the world are faced with unique challenges to their survival, health, and positive development (Hamburg, 1992; Lerner, 1995). For instance, the comorbidity among problem behaviors and the level of youth poverty in the United States have combined to place American youth at unprecedented risk (Jessor, Donovan & Costa, 1991; Ketterlinus & Lamb, 1994; Lerner, 1995; Lerner & Galambos, 1998).

Numerous sectors of society have worked, and continue to work, to address these issues facing youth and the threats to their development. However, although the sum total of these efforts affords a comprehensive approach, the effect on communities has been less than the sum of its parts. Current efforts often involve different agencies and organizations competing for turf, or ownership of a problem, and duplicating services that are delivered independent of input from program recipients. Such an orientation to service provision is quite typically coupled with a deficit view of communities, families, and individuals and, as a consequence, relatively few instances exist of community-wide, integrative collaboration. However, Dryfoos (1998) and Schorr (1997) cite some notable examples of such partnerships. As such, most existing efforts do not identify and then build on community assets and do not create community-based capacity for sustaining effective programs (Benson, 1997; Damon, 1997; Kretzmann & McKnight, 1993; Lerner & Simon, 1998a; McCroskey & Einbinder, 1998).

The profession of family and consumer sciences, formerly known as home economics, came into prominence in the early 1900s to address major societal issues affecting individuals and families (Stage & Vincenti, 1997). For years, home economics was a leading discipline in viewing families and their conditions from an ecological perspective, applying scientific research to address perennial practical problems, and empowering individuals and families to shape their own destinies and that of their communities.

Today, family and consumer sciences, and more broadly the human sciences, along with other disciplines such as psychology, sociology, social work, nursing, and education, utilize an applied developmental science approach. Thus, the community of scholars committed to the use of applied research in relation to human, family, and community well-being has expanded in the latter part of the twentieth century. Focusing on asset-based, community empowerment, these scholars seek to create caring communities through broad and integrative multidisciplinary, multi-professional, multi-institutional, and citizen-led collaborations. They work with schools and communities to design, implement, and evaluate community-based programs. In addition, through scholarship that engages community members in collaborative relationships, the engaged university links programs of proven effectiveness to public policy. Through the education and training of students, applied developmental science programs strive to build a new generation of community leaders dedicated to enhancing the capacity of citizens to use their own and their neighbor's assets and strengths to promote positive development of children and families (e.g., see Benson, 1997; Dryfoos, 1990, 1994, 1998; Hamburg, 1992; Lerner, 1995; Lerner, Ostrom & Freel, 1995, 1997; Ostrom, Lerner & Freel, 1995; Scales & Leffert, 1999; Schorr, 1988, 1997; Weiss & Greene, 1992).

On the one hand, applied developmental scientists, especially those adopting the integrative systems perspective associated with the human sciences (Miller & Lerner, 1994), can collaborate with communities to foster the use of community strengths to pursue valued goals or achieve effective solutions to problems. On the other hand, applied developmental scientists can help insure that communities will have a sustainable source of expertise about programs and policies. Perhaps the key path to such sustainability is education, and scholars may educate their students about ways to engage and influence public policy through partnerships with communities.

HIGHER EDUCATION AND THE PREPARATION OF STUDENTS FOR EFFECTIVE PUBLIC POLICY ENGAGEMENT

A strong democracy is dependent upon enlightened citizens actively participating in their own governance and in the formulation and shaping of public policy. Professionals who work directly or indirectly to enhance the well-being of families need skills to help formulate and shape public policy and to empower individuals and families to actively participate in public policy formation (Brown & Paolucci, 1979). Moreover, professionals need skills in helping individuals and families explore more than one side of an issue using research as a base.

Colleagues involved in the education of scholars and practitioners who will seek to make such contributions have several responsibilities. It is important that they prepare undergraduate and graduate students who understand public policy formation; accept the responsibility to provide leadership and help shape public policy; have the skills needed to effectively engage in public policy formation; understand the role of building effective and appropriately scaled community-based and community-owned programs, ones that integrate community strengths and provide a compelling basis for leveraging public policy; and are concerned with ethical considerations in public policy development.

This education will need to be embedded in the context of several realities:

1. The higher education system, wherein, for instance, basic research and disciplinary education compete for resources with multidisciplinary and multi-professional research and training;
2. The variation in the assets of the diverse communities with which universities may work, and the important racial, ethnic, religious, and cultural differences that may exist in and across these communities; and
3. The public policy arena, wherein politics and the need for action are often at odds with the orientation in universities for reflection and painstaking research.

A focus on understanding these multiple dimensions of reality will be critical to include in the education of professionals aspiring to engage the contemporary policymaking community. Public policy discussions are increasingly directed to placing greater authority and/or autonomy at the state level. As such, state, county, and municipal governments will need to rely on their state and/or local universities for the knowledge applications (e.g., needs assessments, technical assistance, consultations, demonstration projects, and evaluation research) that will be required for the formation of state public policies pertinent to human development.

However, higher education faces several challenges that must be addressed if we are to prepare new professionals for such engagement in the public policy process. First, there is a perception within many of the sectors of the public that we serve that universities are largely disengaged from the problems of everyday life facing the citizens of the communities within their states. Second, there is the perception higher education has not completely fulfilled its implicit, or in some cases explicit, contract to contribute to the public good and to civil society (Boyer, 1994; Kennedy, in press; Spanier, 1997, in press). Third, there is a growing public concern related to access, accountability, and affordability. This concern manifests itself through legislative bodies attempting to exert greater control over policy development for higher education (Boyer, 1994; Magrath, 1998).

Administrative leaders in higher education often articulate appreciation of the service mission of their institutions. However, such statements are often contradicted by internal policies, including promotion and tenure criteria and funding allocations. These policies in fact discourage faculty from the pursuit and application of knowledge to enhance the lives of youth and their families in ways defined by the community as important and valuable (Lerner, 1995; Lerner & Simon, 1998b). Advancing public policy engagement, which links scholarship in teaching and research to service, will require visionary and committed leadership at all administrative levels. Our vision of scholarship insists that "applied" is as important to the intellectual vitality of academe as is "basic" research (Boyer, 1990, 1994; Lerner & Simon, 1998a).

We believe that academic administrative leadership coupled with the legitimization of the scholarship of engagement (Boyer, 1990), or of what has been termed "outreach scholarship" (Lerner, 1995; Lerner & Miller, 1998; Lerner & Simon, 1998b), will result in universities making a more meaningful impact on society. "Outreach," originally pioneered by the USDA Cooperative Extension Service (involving agriculture and home economics), involves using university scholarly expertise for the benefit of audiences and stakeholders external to the university (Lerner & Simon, 1998b; Spanier, 1997, in press; Votruba, 1992, 1996). The concept of outreach scholarship (Lerner, 1995b; Lerner & Simon, 1998b) builds on Boyer's (1990, 1994) notion of the scholarship of engagement and his vision for the "new American college."

Universities are in the knowledge business, that is, they generate, transmit, preserve, or apply knowledge (e.g., in regard to their contributions to their research, teaching, and service missions). Outreach scholarship occurs when universities engage in these knowledge functions to address issues defined by community collaborators as important and/or to attain goals designated as valuable by these community partners. Outreach scholarship occurs, then, in the context of a co-learning association between the university and its community partners, collaborations that require that each partner learn about and accommodate to the other's culture and accept the expertise that each brings to the collaboration. Such scholarship may take the form of asset mapping, needs assessment, issues identification, demonstration research, participatory action research, program design and evaluation, technical assistance (e.g., in grantsmanship or in data base management), and continuing education and training.

Outreach scholarship allows leaders of higher education to integrate the pressures on universities to provide access and accountability to communities with the good will and motivations of faculty to provide service, and to do so in a manner that has currency in the scholarly arena. We believe that the scholarship in applied developmental science provides an exemplary instance of outreach scholarship that serves this integrative role.

THE CONTRIBUTION OF APPLIED DEVELOPMENTAL SCIENCE

The contributions of this book derive from past scholarship pertinent to applied developmental science. As it has been conceptualized by the members of the National Task Force on Applied Developmental Science, applied developmental science (ADS) scholarship represents:

> . . . the programmatic synthesis of research and applications to describe, explain, intervene, and provide preventive and enhancing uses of knowledge about human development. . . . [It is] *applied* [because it has] direct implications for what individuals, practitioners, and policy makers do. . . . [It is] *developmental* [because it] focuses on systematic and successive changes within human systems that occur across the life span. [It is] *science* [because it is] grounded in a range of research methods designed to collect reliable and objective information that can be used to test the validity of theory and applications. (Fisher, et al., 1993, p. 4)

In 1990, in response to the shifting focus of developmental science toward applied issues, the National Task Force on Applied Developmental Science was formed, sponsored by seven national organizations concerned with the promotion of human development at different points along the life span. These organizations were the American Psychological Association, the Society for Research in Child Development, the Society for Research on Adolescence, the National Council on Family Relations, the National Black Child Development Institute, the Gerontological Society of America, and the International Society for Infant Studies. The disciplines represented by these associations have moved toward the ecological and applied science perspective pioneered eighty years earlier by the home economics field. The task force, chaired by Celia Fisher (Fordham University) and John Murray (Kansas State University), was formed to organize the first national conference on graduate education in applied developmental science and to guide future endeavors. Major financial support for the conference was provided by the Foundation for Child Development and the William T. Grant Foundation. On October 10-12, 1991, over fifty leading developmental scientists met at Fordham University to produce a living document that would outline the curriculum and field experiences required to train applied developmental scientists to work with practitioners, social service agencies, and policy makers in the creation of programs that would promote the development of individuals and families (Fisher, et al., 1993).

The conference participants adopted an applied developmental science orientation defined in terms of the above-noted three conjoint aspects (from Fisher, et al., 1993, p. 4). The convergence of these three aspects led to the identification of the reciprocal relationship between theory and application as a cornerstone of applied developmental science, one wherein empirically-based theory not only guides intervention strategies but also is influenced by the outcome of these interventions. Of equal import was the assumption that valid applications of the developmental science base depend upon recognition of the reciprocal nature of person-environment interactions, the influence of individual and cultural diversity on development, an understanding of both normative and atypical developmental processes, and a multidisciplinary perspective aimed at integrating information and skills drawn from relevant biological, social, and behavioral science disciplines.

On September 8-10, 1994, the National Task Force on Applied Developmental Science held a second meeting, hosted by Michigan State University. The meeting was designed to extend the recommendations of the first National Conference to the specific endeavors of applied developmental science programs seeking to produce sustainable university-community partnerships, that is collaborations aimed at delivering "practical" approaches to promoting the development of individuals and families, and the communities in which they live. Representatives of twelve (12) universities with established applied developmental science programs discussed establishing an Inter-University Consortium (IUC) in Applied Developmental Science, one that would develop research and training models of university-community partnerships aimed at enhancing human development. The universities involved in this conference were: Fordham University, Johns Hopkins University, Kansas State University, University of Kansas, University of Maryland, University of Maryland-Baltimore, Michigan State University, University of Michigan, University of Minnesota, University of Nebraska-Lincoln, University of Pennsylvania, and the Pennsylvania State University,

The aspiration of the conference participants was to begin a programmatic multi-site effort which would facilitate the sharing of professional resources to facilitate and support outreach scholarship and policy engagement; the provision to students, faculty, and community collaborators of enhanced training and experience in the knowledge and techniques of applied developmental science; and the reconfiguration of the academy of the future into one in which university reward systems are aligned, through applied developmental science, with the work of scholars and with the needs of the community. Moreover, after the conference, several other universities joined the effort to form a consortium: Florida A & M University, Florida State University, University of Florida, University of Illinois, University of South Florida, and Virginia Polytechnic Institute and State University.

The second conference also resulted in several other important products: 1) The preparation of a special section of the *Journal of Research on Adolescence* (which appeared in 1996) devoted to community-university collaborations promoting positive youth development; 2) The development of an edited book (Lerner & Simon, 1998a) describing the efforts of various public and private universities to foster community-university collaborations aimed at enhancing the life chances of America's youth and families; 3) The initial development of an Applied Developmental Science Outreach-Research Network, a partnership envisioned to (a) provide theoretical advances regarding principles of person-context/relations; (b) develop methods of community collaborative developmental research; (c) identify components of "best practice;" and (d) provide community-collaborative training for a new generation of ADS scholars; and 4) The launching of a new, scholarly vehicle for the dissemination of ADS research, the journal *Applied Developmental Science* (which has been published by Lawrence Erlbaum Associates since January 1997). Richard M. Lerner (Tufts University), Celia B. Fisher (Fordham University), and Richard A. Weinberg (University of Minnesota), are the editors of the journal.

Together, the accomplishments and plans deriving from the Second ADS National Conference have the promise of creating a Zeitgeist for a new model of universities in the twenty-first century. We believe that community-university collaborations involving the applied developmental science approach to outreach scholarship can provide an innovative, value-added contribution of universities to the lives of America's diverse youth, families, and communities. We believe that the probability of this outcome is furthered by the present volume, the result of the Third National ADS conference, which was co-sponsored by the American Association of Family and Consumer Sciences Higher Education Unit (AAFCS-HEU), the Association of Administrators of Human Sciences (AAHS), the National Task Force on Applied Developmental Science, and the Family Institute in the College of Human Sciences at Florida State University, along with other academic units at the university. The means through which this contribution is made derives from the work of the colleagues represented in this volume. A summary of the organization of this book enables this contribution to be specified.

THE PLAN OF THIS BOOK

The goal of the present volume is to advance knowledge about two ways that scholars may foster community partnerships and influence public policies serving youth and families. First, the contributors to this volume seek to specify the dimensions of training and community experience that should be included in educating students to serve communities through the application of developmental science in regard to community-based program development and to public policy engagement. In the section on *Dimensions of Training and Community Collaborations*, authors discuss the features of undergraduate education that are required to prepare undergraduate students to enter emerging roles in communities, ones wherein knowledge about and skills in collaboration and policy engagement will be needed. In turn, authors specify the components of graduate education involved in becoming part of a cadre of professionals providing collaborative and policy engagement leadership in universities, in communities, or in coalitions linking universities and communities. To develop the new professionals needed to promote community partnerships and to engage public policy, the curricula envisioned by authors must prepare students to effectively engage in public policy development regardless of their professional practice arena, be it business, industry, education, government, or human service work.

Moreover, authors contributing to this section stress that classroom-based education is clearly not sufficient to create competent applied developmental scientists. Too often students complete their education with little understanding of, and no experience with, the impact of public policy on their own academic field, careers, and families. Accordingly, authors discuss the types of practicum experiences requisite for education in applied developmental science; chapters in this section illustrate the importance for knowledge development and skill building of experiential learning—in community sites in general and in policy settings in particular. As with any developmental approach to experiential learning, faculty can design an incremental approach to the integration of public policy education and experience into the curriculum. One role of faculty, in conjunction with policy makers, is to determine the logical sequence of education and experiences for students. Thus, the chapters in this section discuss engaging policy makers in the process of developing appropriate practica and internships, ones that involve students in the application of knowledge to specific public policy issues. These experiences, integrated with coursework throughout a degree program, would be aimed at preparing students for the development of community-based solutions, for work with diverse target audiences, and for the evaluation of policy impacts at the individual, community, state, and national levels.

Critical to the success of this training process is the direct involvement of policy makers, community-based professionals, and program participants in the design of the learning experiences students would encounter in the community programs in which they participated. These groups could develop position descriptions for internships and practica; assess and place interns and practicum participants; and continuously evaluate the success of students and the program as a whole. Accordingly, authors discuss the organization of these activities, one that engages a university system transformed to promote collaborations with communities. Finally, then, the general features of successful partnerships between communities and universities in regard to program development and policy engagement are discussed, and examples are provided of actual partnerships that continue to provide a context for student training and a resource to communities.

However, while there are validated ideas about curricular development for undergraduate and graduate students, and instances of successful university-community collaborations involving the faculty of and the students in such educational programs, there is still much to be learned about building effective and sustained links among universities, communities, and policy makers. These linkages are still relatively new in academe and, often, obstacles occur in trying to initiate and sustain such efforts. Certainly, the differences among the cultures of the university, the community, and policy makers provide formidable challenges to collaborations. Institutions having a core purpose of reflection and knowledge generation, transmission, preservation, and application (Boyer, 1990, 1994), differ from those having a service utilization and advocacy orientation. Both of these types of institutions are different from those that deliver services within the context of political pressures.

These cultural differences are discussed in several of the chapters in the section of this book on *Contemporary Challenges: Community and University Perspectives*. Representatives of all components of the envisioned university-community-policymaking linkage share a belief in the usefulness of collaboration, in involving the university in service to the community through its educational and research missions, and in learning about the perspectives of all partners in order to enhance and sustain the linkage. However, given their institution's different functions and the contrasting cultural values and attitudes associated with them, the authors in this section make clear that the perspectives of leaders in state government, in the world of community-based, non-governmental organizations (NGOs), and in the university are not isomorphic. Simply, the political, action/advocacy, and reflective character of these three components of the envisioned linkage, respectively, contribute to the cultural differences that must be understood and—in order for partnerships to be effective—overcome.

Moreover, the chapters in this section make clear that there is important cultural variation *within* universities. It is certainly the case that cultural (e.g., value and attitudinal) differences exist in the policy making community (e.g., across the political spectrum involved with the two major political parties) and in the NGO/not-for-profit community (e.g., in regard to approaches that advocate for policies in general versus those that work to generate funding for particular service delivery). However, these cultural differences are often well known to the public (e.g., as is the case in regard to the different perspectives of political parties) and, in any case, are readily accessible (e.g., through media coverage).

The culture of the university is less well-known to the community. Indeed, keeping the culture of the university apart from the community has been a defining feature of higher education throughout almost all of the twentieth century. The development of this nation's system of higher education has involved the elaboration within America of the nineteenth-century German model of a university as an institution disengaged from the ebb and flow of the mundane issues confronting the society around it; such a university, through its faculty, was free to pursue "pure" (ethereal) knowledge in a manner unconstrained (or, perhaps better, uncontaminated) by a society focused on the concrete problems of everyday life (Bonnen, 1998; Boyer, 1990; Lynton & Elman, 1987). In America, those faculty best able to pursue ethereal knowledge were the most highly regarded and the most rewarded within their institutions, and—perhaps associated as well with the American ethos of rugged individualism—a university culture emerged wherein independent scholarly productivity by a faculty member in the development of basic knowledge was the ideal academic profile (Awbrey, Scott & Vincenti, 1997; Bok, 1982, 1990, 1992).

Given this history, universities, if they are to become institutions collaborating with communities and government in the service of children and their families, and if they are to train a new generation of professionals aiding and leading such multi-sector collaborations, have a special burden to reveal clearly the nature of their culture. University leaders must present to the community the cultural variation that exists currently within higher education regarding—most centrally—a commitment to community involvement and collaboration (Lerner, 1995); and they must provide access to the community to participate in the debates now occurring in academe about increasing this commitment (Bok, 1982, 1990, 1992; Richardson, 1996; Spanier, 1997, in press). They must overcome the deserved skepticism within the community about the seriousness of the commitment of universities to collaborate in a sustained manner and to use their knowledge resources to add value, in community-defined ways, to the lives of children and families.

The chapters in the *Contemporary Challenges* section underscore this cultural variation within the university and the tasks involved in creating openness and engagement that lie ahead. In addition, the chapters delineate the different orientations toward and roles of faculty, of colleges or schools, and of central administration in addressing these challenges. Moreover, a final set of chapters in this section provides voice to the ideas of the philanthropic community about the potential for applied developmental science serving the vision of communities regarding children and families. In addition, however, these chapters underscore the continued skepticism that foundation leaders have about whether the university—as an institution—can undergo sufficient cultural change to actualize research and education agendas that effectively and sustainably serve the community and engage policy makers.

Clearly, a new action agenda is required if universities are to become effectively engaged as institutions to work with communities to bring about desired social change and to educate professionals to become leaders for healthy individuals, families, and communities. The afterwords that follow the *Contemporary Challenges* section offer visions for such action and the appendices present a compendium of ideas about what serves as action agendas for transforming the university.

In sum, then, this book seeks to link universities, communities, and policy makers in the service of our nation's families and individuals. We believe that this linkage is vital for the enhancement of the lives of the individuals and families of the communities of our nation. More generally, we believe that the scholarship presented in this book adds importantly to the ongoing discussion (Bok, 1990; Boyer, 1990, 1994; Kennedy, in press; Richardson, 1996; Spanier, 1997, in press) of the potential role that universities can play in furthering civil society in America.

CONCLUSIONS

We believe that this book offers a useful frame for multi-disciplinary and multi-organizational partnerships involving the training of a new generation of professionals, individuals able to integrate scholarship, policy engagement, and service.   Through the leadership of the American Association of Family and Consumer Sciences (AAFCS), the Association of Administrators of Human Sciences (AAHS), and the National ADS Task Force, we hope that this book will engage the interest of other scholarly and professional organizations in collaborating to develop a new generation of professionals with public policy interests and engagement skills.

Such an integration of education and public policy constitutes a unique, significant, and timely contribution to civil society in America. We will be pleased if this book helps to launch a discussion of standards for public policy education, one that will impact the careers of future professionals prepared in the human development sciences as well as in other related fields of study. Such a synthesis of expertise, combined with a commitment to serve through knowledge, will be an indisputable value-added contribution of universities to enhancing the quality of life of America's children and families.

REFERENCES

Awbrey, S., Scott, D. & Vincenti, V. (1997). Transformation of the university: Implications for teaching. In P. Ralston & V. Vincenti (Eds.), *Teaching in land-grant and state universities: New perspectives in human sciences.* Washington, DC: National Association of State Universities and Land-Grant Colleges.

Benson, P. (1997). *All kids are our kids: What communities must do to raise caring and responsible children and adolescents.* San Francisco: Jossey-Bass.

Bok, D. (1982). *Beyond the ivory tower: Social responsibilities of the modern university.* Cambridge, MA: Harvard University Press.

Bok, D. (1990). *Universities and the future of America.* Durham, NC: Duke University Press.

Bok, D. (1992, July/August). Reclaiming the public trust. *Change,* 13-19.

Boyer, E. L. (1990). *Scholarship reconsidered: Priorities of the professoriate.* Princeton, NJ: The Carnegie Foundation for the Advancement of Teaching.

Boyer, E. L. (1994, March 9). Creating the new American college. *The Chronicle of Higher Education,* A48.

Brown, M. & Paolucci, B. (1979). *Home economics: A definition.* Washington, DC: American Home Economics Association.

Damon, W. (1997). *The youth charter: How communities can work together to raise standards for all our children.* New York: The Free Press.

Dryfoos, J. G. (1990). *Adolescents at risk: Prevalence and prevention.* New York: Oxford University Press.

Dryfoos, J. G. (1994). *Full service schools: A revolution in health and social services for children, youth, and families.* San Francisco: Jossey-Bass.

Dryfoos, J. G. (1998). *Safe passage: Making it through adolescence in a risky society.* New York: Oxford University Press.

Fisher, C. B., Murray, J. P., Dill, J. R., Hagen, J. W., Hogan, M. J., Lerner, R. M., Rebok, G. W., Sigel, I., Sostek, A. M., Smyer, M. A., Spencer, M. B. & Wilcox, B. (1993). The national conference on graduate education in the applications of developmental science across the life-span. *Journal of Applied Developmental Psychology, 14,* 1-10.

Hamburg, D. A. (1992). *Today's children: Creating a future for a generation in crisis.* New York: Time Books.

Kennedy, E. M. (in press). University-community partnerships: A mutually beneficial effort to aid community development and improve academic learning opportunities. *Applied Developmental Science.*

Ketterlinus, R. D. & Lamb, M. E. (Eds.). (1994). *Adolescent problem behaviors: Issues and research.* Hillsdale, NJ: Erlbaum.

Kretzmann, J. P. & McKnight, J. L. (1993). *Building communities from the inside out: A path towards finding and mobilizing a community's assets.* Chicago, IL: ACTA Publications.

Lerner, R. M. (1995). *America's youth in crisis: Challenges and options for programs and policies.* Thousand Oaks, CA: Sage.

Lerner, R. M. & Galambos, N. L. (1998). Adolescent development: Challenges and opportunities for research, programs, and policies. In J. T. Spence (Ed.), *Annual Review of Psychology* (Vol. 49, pp. 413-446). Palo Alto, CA: Annual Reviews.

Lerner, R. M., Ostrom, C. W. & Freel, M. A. (1995). Promoting positive youth and community development through outreach scholarship: Comments on Zeldin and Peterson. *Journal of Adolescent Research, 10,* 486-502.

Lerner, R. M., Ostrom, C. W. & Freel, M. A. (1997). Preventing health compromising behaviors among youth and promoting their positive development: A developmental contextual perspective. In J. Schulenberg, J. L. Maggs & K. Hurrelmann (Eds.), *Health risks and developmental transitions during adolescence* (pp. 498-521). New York: Cambridge University Press.

Lerner, R. M. & Miller, J. M. (1998). Developing multidisciplinary institutes to enhance the lives of individuals and families: Academic potentials and pitfalls. *Journal of Public Service and Outreach, 3*(1), 64-73.

Lerner, R. M. & Simon, L. A. K. (1998a). The new American outreach university: Challenges and options. In R. M. Lerner & L. A. K. Simon (Eds.), *University-community collaborations for the twenty-first century: Outreach scholarship for youth and families* (pp. 3-23). New York: Garland.

Lerner, R. M. & Simon, L. A. K. (Eds.). (1998b). *University-community collaborations for the twenty-first century: Outreach scholarship for youth and families.* New York: Garland.

Lynton, E. A. & Elman, S. E. (1987). *New priorities for the university: Meeting society's needs for applied knowledge and competent individuals.* San Francisco: Jossey-Bass.

Magrath, C. P. (1998). Foreword: Creating a new outreach university. In R. M. Lerner & L. A. K. Simon (Eds.), *University-community collaborations for the twenty-first century: Outreach scholarship for youth and families* (pp. xiii-xx). New York: Garland.

McCroskey, J. & Einbinder, S. D. (Eds.). (1998). *Universities and communities: Remaking professional and interprofessional education for the next century.* Westport, CT: Greenwood Press.

Miller, J. M. & Lerner, R. M. (1994). Integrating research and outreach: Developmental contextualism and the human ecological perspective. *Home Economics Forum, 7,* 21-28.

Ostrom, C. W., Lerner, R. M. & Freel, M. A. (1995). Building the capacity of youth and families through university-community collaborations: The development-in-context evaluation (DICE) model. *Journal of Adolescent Research, 10,* 427-448.

Richardson, W.C. (1996). *A new calling for higher education.* The John W. Olswald Lecture. University Park, PA: The Pennsylvania State University.

Scales, P. & Leffert, N. (1999). *Developmental assets: A synthesis of the scientific research on adolescent development.* Minneapolis, MN: Search Institute.

Schorr, L. B. (1988). *Within our reach: Breaking the cycle of disadvantage.* New York: Doubleday.

Schorr, L. B. (1997). *Common purpose: Strengthening families and neighborhoods to rebuild America.* New York: Doubleday.

Spanier, G.B. (1997). *Enhancing the quality of life for children, youth, and families.* Unpublished manuscript. University Park, PA: The Pennsylvania State University.

Spanier, G. B. (in press). Enhancing the quality of life: A model for the 21st century land-grant university. *Applied Developmental Science.*

Stage, S. & Vincenti, V. (Eds.). (1997). *Rethinking home economics: Women and the history of a profession.* Ithaca, NY: Cornell University Press.

Weiss, H. B. & Greene, J. C. (1992). An empowerment partnership for family support and education programs and evaluations. *Family Science Review, 5,* 131-148.

The Future of Public Policy Engagement: Preparing Human Sciences Undergraduates for Emerging Roles

Connie Ley, *Illinois State University*

In the 21st century, the vast majority of bachelor's degree recipients in the human sciences[1] will be on the front-line working most directly with family issues and implementing policies that affect families. They will work with the steadily increasing numbers of children who live in families that have no fathers or in families that have no homes. They will serve individuals and families who face and will continue to face the ever increasingly complex challenges which the future holds. These novice professionals also will be asked to work in new ways to meet the needs of the clients they serve. Involvement with public policy will be a critical role for human sciences experts in serving families and the profession. While innumerable scholars have suggested what policies and foci are essential for the work of human sciences professionals (e.g., Fine, 1992; Jenson & Warstadt, 1990; Kellett, 1994; Wisensale, 1992; Zimmerman, 1992), fewer experts have addressed the means by which professionals are to gain levels of expertise to effectively engage in the public policy arena.

What processes, attitudes or attributes, knowledge and skills should undergraduates in applied developmental science fields acquire which will make them effective in engaging in politics? That is, politics as described by David Mathews in his book *Politics for People* (1994), in which he simply says politics is fostering the well-being of the community by public action. This public action is represented by a wide range of formal and informal efforts to solve common problems and advance the common well-being of community members. In determining how to educate best undergraduates for roles in the public policy/political arena[2], it is imperative to think of politics more broadly than the strict traditional sense such as politics dominated by politicians, lobbyists and bureaucracies. A definition of political activity must include citizen politics which is commonly manifested in neighborhood associations, public forums and other such grassroots groups. Professionals require a set of competencies which provides the ability to function appropriately in the traditional political arena and the capacity to achieve civic action through the realm of citizen politics. With this in mind the following assumptions become essential concepts regarding public policy education for human sciences professionals:

- Hold a broader view of public policy development including those actions which affect public well-being that are developed in board rooms of businesses and not-for-profit organizations where human sciences professionals may work.
- Understand that one type of political activity cannot substitute or compensate for another; one type is not good and another bad.

- Are competent in the myriad political environments which exist now and will emerge in the future. Graduates should gain the leadership capacity for bringing the actions of these various realms into congruence.

Coupled with this broad view of public policy arenas is the comprehensive view of human sciences professions. Individuals educated as human sciences experts include those who study life cycle human development and those with expertise in family resource development, management and utilization (i.e., experts in apparel and textiles, family economics, food and nutrition, and housing and environmental design). These professionals find themselves in businesses, governmental and nongovernmental social service agencies, and other not-for-profit organizations which contribute to human well-being. In these settings, human development professionals can play important decision-making roles regarding life-affecting activities, products, and services offered by these employing organizations.

This chapter proposes a framework for the undergraduate curricula in fields of applied developmental science. These are guidelines for preparing aspiring professionals for activity in the public policy arena. The ideas presented here are based on past experiences and current literature. Several caveats are noted. This framework should not be viewed as complete. It is presented as a springboard for professional dialogue focusing on the public policy/political expertise needed by persons who complete baccalaureate degrees in applied developmental science.

BACKGROUND

Several themes dominate the literature about government and public policy involvement. These themes are nonpartisan, pervade the continuum of the political spectrum from liberal to conservative, and are touted by practitioners and scholars. Lappé and DuBois (1994, p. xiii) refer to it as "living democracy," a new stage in our democratic system. Osborne and Gaebler (1992, p. xix) use the term "entrepreneurial government," to describe what they say is on the rise across our country. Mathews (1994, p. 121) under the auspices of the Harwood Group use the phrase, "Politics that is not called politics," to describe what people say about their own public participation to create a community and a life that addresses issues and inequities, but is not politics! Even in the realm of public management/ administration what some might construe as the staunchly impenetrable bureaucracy itself comes a new beam of light. Some reports from public administration (Lynn, 1996; Kettl, Ingraham, Sanders & Horner, 1996) use terminology such as breaking bureaucracy, reinventing government, replacement of hierarchical control and other ideas which are a marked departure from traditional thinking in this field. In the public policy arena where issues are so often divided, it is important to pay attention to those areas where agreement seems to have occurred serendipitously.

A report, *Civil Service Reform*, from the Brookings Institution affords insights about proposed directions for the bureaucratic system. Kettl, et al. (1996) suggest the importance of conflict management as essential for public sector employees who will be faced with the task of refereeing among groups with generational, geographic, cultural and myriad other divergent interests. These analysts indicate that scarce resources will be used to create, store, retrieve, integrate and apply knowledge about service delivery for the public, in contrast to the current system in which they say resources are spent to maintain hierarchical control. The increasing decentralization will create less need for system managers and more need for information managers and integrators.

Kettl, et al. (1996) discuss a phenomenon which is readily apparent to nongovernmental agencies and organizations as well, that is the ever increasing interdependence on creating partnerships and collaborative arrangements to solve problems. They describe the need to move from narrowly controlling programs to solving problems that hinder partnerships. There is a long road to overcoming government management systems and the civil service system which do not lend themselves to this type of operation. Kellett (1994) accentuated a similar message when she stressed the imperative for professionals to act collaboratively on behalf of families. If human sciences professionals can enter the workplace where many will work in government-related situations and have the skills needed to change the system, they may find themselves in leadership roles creating new governmental policies and procedures for service delivery.

Kettl, et al. (1996) also describe a changing political architecture which will alter the modes of citizen access to and participation in government. This will result in some respects because distinctions between the public and private sectors will be blurred. Increasingly technology will allow people to participate much more directly in their own governance. To revitalize itself, the civil service system will need to hire new workers and train current workers with negotiation skills, leadership ability, a sense of global thinking, positive attitudes about flexible work environments, and skills to allow them to respond to the increasing need for accountability. Kettl, et al. describe what civil servants of the future should be like.

> Government will need policy specialists who are functional generalists. From public health systems . . . to environmental puzzles . . . tough problems will bedevil policy makers. Government will need its own expertise to sort through claims about the sources and solutions to these problems. The problems will not respect organizational boundaries, so the governments institutional memory experts will need to cross these boundaries in their careers and in their thinking. Most important, these experts will need to provide the government with intelligence to digest and interpret the information that flows in from the government's partners. No private company will dream of shaping critical policies based on data solely supplied by those trying to sell it something. Government needs to be just as smart. (p. 75)

Other authors emphasize ideas relative to political engagement. Anderson and Miles (1990) indicate that public policy is derived in the public and private sectors. They note that as families interact with businesses, communities, governments and other families (who in turn are linked to other families, businesses, communities and governments globally), the persistent dilemmas of families manifest themselves with more complexity. Anderson and Miles highlight the Cooperative Extension activities of the land-grant system, but the functions of public policy education they describe are applicable to any applied developmental science professionals regardless of the setting in which they practice. The concepts they highlight include knowing the issue analysis process, knowing how to educate "supporting participants" (the public, colleagues, bosses, and politicians) about issue analysis and various political engagement processes, and knowing how to test strategies.

Lappé and DuBois (1994) suggest both one-on-one skills and group skills which are practical tools for their "living democracy." Although these are defined as skills for all citizens, human sciences professionals need these skills and must be able to convey them to clients and others. The proficiencies they emphasize are active listening, creative conflict, mediation, negotiation, political imagination, public dialogue, public judgment, celebration and appreciation, evaluation and reflection and mentoring. Lappé and DuBois call these arts of democracy.

Viewing political expertise as art is not unique to Lappé and DuBois. Lynn (1996) uses the term art in the title of his book, *Public Management as Art, Science and Profession*. He attempts to untangle the concerns about public management which he says is an amalgam of public policy and public administration. As he sorts through the scholar and practitioner concerns regarding his field, he defines some functions of public managers as art. Lynn reaffirms the ideas put forth by several other authors regarding the need for new ways of thinking about accomplishing public policy agendas. He portrays the effective public administrator in the future as one who works to establish coalitions, communicates effectively with a variety of audiences, and can see the broad scope of questions which must be addressed by policy makers. His concern for public administrators who must move through the bureaucratic maze is evident in his writing.

Osborne and Gaebler (1994) take a different approach in their view of public policy. In fact, they have been criticized by some colleagues for viewing government, public policy and the bureaucracy with a business perspective. They suggest government take on an entrepreneurial attitude as it provides services, develops policies, and addresses citizen and community needs. Their ideas include encouraging healthy competition, empowering clients/citizens, focusing on accomplishing outcomes, and being mission driven rather than a slave to rules and regulations. In addition, they say entrepreneurs prevent problems rather than provide services to fix problems, operate in a decentralized mode, embrace participatory management and build coalitions.

Family and consumer sciences professionals have a proud of history of public policy involvement as described by Meszaros and Cummings (1983). In the 1980s home economics scholars examined the socialization and participation patterns of home economics professionals (Cummings, 1982; Cummings & Hirschlein, 1984; Ley, 1980, 1982; Neruda, 1979; Sheehan & Vaughn, 1991; Tripple, 1990; and Vickers, 1985). Research done by Ley (1980) suggested that experiences with political issues and public figures encouraged participation. She proposed a process as the means to increasing political activity among home economics professionals. Her plan included such methods as developing a rationale for involvement; gaining confidence, skill and experience; and participating in actual engagement activities (Ley, 1982).

Vickers (1985) augmented Ley's ideas on effective public policy. She proposed one way of gaining confidence would be to participate in policy decision-making on the job. Evaluation of policies, product development, curriculum decisions were used as examples of policy-related activities home economists engaged in on-the-job. Laab (1994) talked more broadly about women influencing policies at work by suggesting that being active in policy formation can contribute to overall career advancement. Vickers also explained another way of gaining confidence might be to engage in public affairs training. Tripple (1990) presented a model for political socialization to prepare students for advocacy roles and provide a level of confidence for entering the public policy arena. Cummings (1982) reported that college and university faculty who believed home economists should be politically active said that political activities and skill building are appropriate objectives for undergraduate majors in home economics. The premise here is that politically active professionals will work toward socializing the next generation of human sciences professionals.

Throughout the literature on public policy involvement there is reference to terms such as advocacy, empowerment, lobbying, prevention, and other possible politically related actions. It is essential that professionals in applied developmental science know what these various activities encompass. Perhaps even more consequential is the ability to judge the appropriate professional involvement in a specific situation.

To make the determination regarding appropriate political involvement, sound judgment is essential. In *Human Judgment and Social Policy*, Hammond (1996) suggests an approach to policy formation which is different from the usual opinion held by policy analysts. Traditionally, students of policy formation focus on the content of various policies. Hammond's focuses on cognitive process or the judgments by which social policies are created. Efforts to educate students about public policy formation should highlight the development of policies which help to level the playing field rather than prescribe outcomes. Hammond's view lends itself well to this perspective.

> . . . the policy maker's task of integrating scientific information into the fabric of social values is an extraordinarily difficult task for which there is no textbook, no handbook, no operating manual, no equipment, no set of heuristics, no history, not even a tradition— unless a record of confusion can be called a tradition. Young scientists learning their trade will have all the advantages, all of those supports for successful cognition. Young artists are accorded at least some appreciation for the difficulties of their creative efforts. But young policymakers learning their trade have none of these supporters; each effort to integrate scientific facts and social values starts fresh, as if it had never been attempted before. (p. 264-265)

Professionals in human sciences know all too well this challenge to synthesize knowledge which Hammond underscores. In his book he reviews the study of correspondence and coherence judgment. At the risk of being too simplistic, these two types of thinking might be defined as follows. Coherence judgments are empirically based requiring a sound grasp of statistics and data interpretation. Correspondence judgment is rooted in the range and types of experiences found in ones history of living. Students preparing for careers in applied developmental science must achieve competence in both forms of judgment. The challenge for educators is how to develop well-honed coherence thinking along with the more difficult to teach correspondence judgment.

There is another mode of thinking that is essential for public policy involvement. Numerous politicians and political scientists of diverse political persuasions (e.g., Osborne & Gaebler, 1992; Perot & Simon, 1996; Thompson, 1996) tout the importance of common sense government. In the study of cognition judgment common sense is placed near a midpoint on the continuum. "The forms of cognition that lie on the continuum between intuition and analysis. . . . This form of cognition is known to the layperson as common sense" (Hammond, 1996, p. 150).

Is it possible to teach common sense? Hammond (1996) suggests that a wide range of experiences help provide a basis for learning common sense. The assessment of such learning is difficult at best, thus educators may strive to develop common sense in students, but will have difficulty determining a level of accomplishment for this competence.

Professionals who would influence public policy should be proficient ethical leaders. Robert Theobald (1992) relates implications for ethical effectiveness. He suggests that in order to move toward more viable human societies, people need opportunities to learn the value of 1) honesty, responsibility, and compassion; 2) the necessity for learning to live with uncertainty; 3) majority rule and minority rights; 4) socioeconomic equity and social justice; and 5) learning as the impetus for change rather than power. Terry (1993) conveys to his reader that leadership is "to take responsibility for ourselves in concert with others, seeking to create and build a

global commonwealth worthy of the best that we as human beings have to offer."
Each person emerges as a leader at various points in time. Human sciences
professionals are often found in professional situations of leadership as Terry
describes.

Public policy involvement introduces a variety of opportunities to provide
leadership and myriad leadership models exist. Ambrose (1991) relates that leaders
who are authentic, ethical and confident will succeed with influencing those around
them. Her tenets of leadership resonate in reflective human action. The reflective
human action perspective (Andrews, Mitstifer, Rehm, & Vaughn, 1995) may be one
of the most viable for the human sciences profession. Reflective human action has
four essential components: Authenticity, ethical sensibility, spirituality and action.
Andrews and Clark (1996) describe the need for leadership in our profession. "We
are living in a time when professionals must step forward and be able to take
leadership in ways that 'cement' the need for including . . . family and consumer
sciences professionals in work, social and policy issues affecting individuals and
families. The reflective human action model provides an avenue for this type of
leadership" (p. 2).

The unique feature of public policy involvement for human sciences
professionals is the attention given to the complexity of roles and actions which
individuals and families are expected to perform in their daily lives. The dilemmas
precipitated by these everyday occurrences are known as persistent practical
problems (Brown & Paolucci, 1979) and typically manifest themselves in each
generation with distinct characteristics. A strong understanding of these persistent
questions faced by every generation is an essential part of the education for public
policy involvement. Perhaps a mission for applied developmental science could be
adapted from the mission (Brown & Paolucci, 1979) entrusted to home economics:

> to enable families as individual units . . . to build and maintain
> systems of action which lead . . . to enlightened cooperative
> participation with critique and formulation of social goals and the
> means for accomplishing them. (p. 23)

The idea that human sciences professionals should engage, energize and
educate the citizenry is discussed in other sections of this chapter, but it bears
repeating here as the reader is asked to reflect on the statement from Brown and
Paolucci. The task of helping people shape their own destiny through self-
determination, while maintaining a vision of what will benefit the community and
the world at large, is of paramount importance to us all. It is a worthy mission.

Baldwin (1991) suggests that for too long the theoretical knower was separated
from the political actor. To make an impact for families now and in the future, the
roles of specialist scholar and citizen should merge. Scholars in applied
developmental science should make every effort to deftly combine theory and
practice and convey this expectation to students.

ESTABLISHING A CURRICULAR FRAMEWORK

This brief examination of specific literature and the collective experiences and
background of this audience of interested professionals will assist with the
formulation of concepts necessary for provocative and practical education for
public policy involvement. The plan presented here is based on the premise that
learning for public policy engagement involves three learning spheres: Acquisition
of attitudes/attributes, development of expertise with processes and skills, and
mastery of basic information and premises related to public policy. In Figure 2.1

the competencies for the three spheres of learning are depicted. It is important to think of these spheres of learning as interdependent, thus providing an opportunity for students to build a personal system for public policy engagement.

ATTITUDES/ ATTRIBUTES	PROCESS/SKILLS	KNOWLEDGE
Circumstance Acuity	Coalition Building	Change Process
Common Sense	Communication	Comparative Family
Confidence	Conflict Management	Policy
Entrepreneurial	Critical Thinking	Leadership
Thinking	Education/Teaching	Characteristics
Ethical Conduct	Forecasting	Persistent Practical
Leadership	Issue Analysis	Problems/Critical
	Leadership	Family Issues
	Outcomes Assessment	Policymaking Processes
	Policy Analysis	Policymaking Roles for
	Policy Development	Human Sciences
	Research Utilization	Professionals
	Technology	Power Theories
	Applications	Specific Subject Matter

Figure 2.1 Essential Concepts in Three Spheres of Learning for Public Policy
Education in the Human Sciences.

A majority of the competencies suggested are valuable assets for the entire citizenry. It is imperative for professionals in applied developmental science is to be well-grounded in citizen skills. They can then be effective as individuals in the public policy arena and provide leadership and education for others regarding political engagement. It would be naive to assume that undergraduate students will arrive on campus with keen citizenship skills.

One underlying principle which should guide efforts to design curriculum for public policy involvement is that no one course will provide all that is needed. Nor could one course provide the type of educational experience that will create attributes and foster attitudes essential for competent professionals.

The knowledge competencies suggested for this curricular framework include understanding the change process, discerning comparative family policy, analyzing components of leadership, recognizing persistent practical problems and critical family issues, comprehending public and private policymaking processes, recognizing policymaking roles for human sciences professionals, recognizing power structures, and learning subject matter specific knowledge. Knowledge and understanding of these various concepts will be a critical part of the undergraduate curricular framework for public policy education.

Concepts in the knowledge sphere will provide a basis for action. They will contribute to developing the attitudes/attributes, and skills/processes critical to the performance of human sciences professionals. Aside from merely gaining knowledge, "existing knowledge must be examined with the goal of gaining critical distance on what has been absorbed uncritically in school and everyday life" (Shor, 1992, p. 119). Shor calls this experience part of a desocialization process which not only recognizes the need to question existing knowledge, but also sees knowledge and acquisition of knowledge as part of the political process which often emphasizes inclusion and exclusion. He uses the example that, while our daily newspapers routinely include business news, they also routinely exclude labor news. It is a heavy burden on an instructor to take on the task of resocializing our students by presenting a broad knowledge base and also helping students to reconfigure the knowledge they bring to our classes. It is imperative that students' training also create a thirst to this broad knowledge base to insure that they continue to pursue broad knowledge as part of their continuing professional education after graduation.

The notion of knowledge is underscored by Delli Carpini and Keeter (1996) particularly as it relates to political knowledge. They relate an appropriate base of political knowledge to political and socioeconomic power. Knowledge is not only an important political resource in its own right, but also serves as a facilitator to other sources of power.

The largest category of competencies for public policy involvement is found in the skills/processes sphere. In the realm of public policy education for human sciences professionals, efforts to design curriculum must remain cognizant of the fact that young human sciences professionals will not only use these skills and processes themselves, but also will train others to use them. The list is long and, as is true with learning any skill, practice over time will be a deciding factor in the success of an educational plan.

Communication (both oral and written), conflict mediation, education methods (teaching policymakers and public/clients), forecasting (trends for families, for family policies), issue analysis, leadership, outcomes assessment, policy analysis, policy development, problem solving/critical thinking, research utilization, team/coalition building and technology application are some of the most useful processes for the novice professional in human sciences.

Possibly the most complex teaching/learning occurs when trying to formulate attitudes or develop particular individual attributes. Learning in this sphere requires an extended time period to allow for assimilation of experiences which leads to attitude or attribute development. It is also difficult to measure the success of learning in this domain due to the esoteric nature of attitudes and personal qualities. However, the complicated nature of the task at hand does not negate the importance of the acquisition of attitudes and attributes such as circumstance acuity which is an appreciation and sensitivity to diverse responses of diverse people in diverse situations, confidence, common sense, ethical conduct and entrepreneurial thinking which encompasses a list of traits including mission-driven and prevention-oriented.

Learning in each of the spheres will be more effective if students are engaged in active learning—the type of learning which finds students involved directly and intensely in experiences which make knowledge meaningful and provide practice for developing skills and attitudes.

THE CHALLENGE

The challenge then is, how best to prepare undergraduates in human sciences for roles in the public policy arena. Education for public policy involvement at the undergraduate level should permeate the undergraduate curriculum. Designing courses specifically for public policy training and those which integrate public policy concepts into subject matter courses is one fundamental way to foster the needed competencies. A model creating public policy effectiveness includes a scope of learning as illustrated in Figure 2.2. This model is the overview for the broad educational experiences both curricular and extracurricular which would provide training in public policy expertise.

The Overview

General education on local campuses should provide a foundation for public policy competence. Political science, economics, communications, psychology, sociology and other disciplines share a responsibility for laying the groundwork for public

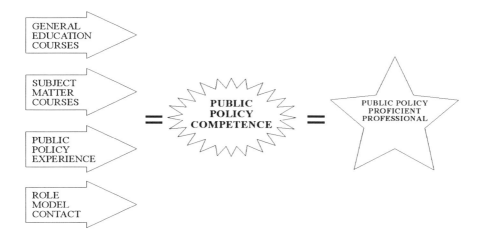

Figure 2.2 Model for Undergraduate Education for Public Policy Involvement.

policy education. University programs in the human sciences must strive to insure the best possible general education curriculum which provides essential building blocks for other essential learning with respect to public policy involvement.

Subject matter courses in the human sciences also will provide the background and expertise which make human sciences professionals unique in their perspective when addressing public policy concerns. A sound education in the knowledge and skills of applied developmental science is one means of insuring a high level of public confidence in the applied developmental science professional. These subject matter courses may also provide a venue for presenting and practicing public policy skills in the context of particular human sciences issues and ideas.

There should also be specific courses to prepare students for public policy involvement. One course will provide the complete learning experience needed for preparing professionals for the complex realm of political engagement. Distinct courses focusing on public policy and the integration of public policy concepts into specific subject matter courses will provide a realistic focus for the types of situations human sciences professionals face.

Students will need actual experiences with public policy situations. Tripple (1990) proposed an advocacy model. She suggested steps for helping students build confidence in the legislative environment. While her model is directed specifically to experiences with legislators, there are a variety of experiences which provide the opportunity for students to see that they can influence the world around them.

One way to give students experience with affecting policies could begin by allowing them to influence course syllabi (the class policies). An instructor might give students an initial draft of the syllabus, including goals, topics, calendar, and projects for the class. Students would review the syllabus and determine whether they feel the design is one which meets their needs. They could propose alternative projects, project due dates, rearrange topics, or other such changes by providing the new idea and an appropriate rationale. Students would have the opportunity to negotiate for the entire class or just for themselves. This experience allows them to observe the instructor providing rebuttals. Through this activity students could find a unique sense of power and confidence in their own ideas. They would have important interactions with stakeholders (other students and the instructor). This example would make influencing policy a very real experience for students.

Realistic public policy experience also encompasses many and frequent opportunities to have contact with role models who are influencing public policy. Faculty members are often in the most immediate environment for students to observe. Often faculty share with students the public policy efforts in which they are involved. Experiences with setting national apparel sizing standards, influencing building codes and standards for housing, nutrition policies, child care advocacy, parenting education, and court mandated divorce mediation are all public policy issues that students on campus have seen faculty undertake. Also, alumni, fellow students, internship supervisors and others provide opportunities for students to see "someone like me" or "someone I aspire to be like" engaging in the public policy arena.

Introducing Public Policy to Human Sciences Students

The introductory course would present the idea of public policy involvement as a professional role and include content and processes to raise student awareness. Figure 2.3 uses the list of competencies presented in Figure 2.1 to illustrate the essential learning for the initial course. However, students would have exposure to the entire list of competencies, thus illustrating the benchmark of performance they are attempting to achieve. To initiate the development of essential attitudes and attributes, an awareness of the need for these traits would be part of the induction rite. The goal is to provide aspiring family and consumer sciences professionals with a sense of importance regarding these traits. Students would be encouraged to begin and maintain a portfolio of their work to demonstrate their development and growth in achieving the necessary competencies.

ATTITUDES/ ATTRIBUTES	PROCESS/SKILLS	KNOWLEDGE
*Circumstance Acuity	*Coalition Building	*Change Process*
*Common Sense	*Communication	*Comparative Family*
*Confidence	*Conflict Management*	*Policy*
*Entrepreneurial	*Critical Thinking	*Leadership
Thinking	*Education/Teaching	Characteristics
*Ethical Conduct	*Forecasting*	*Persistent Practical
	Issue Analysis	Problems/Critical
	*Leadership	Family Issues
	Outcomes Assessment	*Policymaking
	*Policy Analysis	Processes
	*Policy Development	*Policymaking Roles
	*Research Utilization	for Human
	*Technology	Sciences
	Applications	Professionals
		Power Theories
		Specific Subject Matter

Figure 2.3 Identification of Competencies for an Introductory Course in Public
Policy Involvement.

* indicates those concepts emphasized in an introductory course in public policy involvement
Italicized words indicate those concepts to be included in public policy courses beyond the *introductory level.*

Knowledge of persistent practical problems and how they manifest themselves as critical family issues will be part of this course and reinforced throughout the collegiate career. An understanding of this concept will provide a basis for the importance of specific subject matter knowledge which will be the focus of a large portion of the undergraduate students' coursework. Students would also be acquainted with the policymaking role of human sciences professionals and the process by which public policies are made. All of these concepts will be a cornerstones of this introductory course.

Process and skill development will also begin at this level as well. The class should give students experiences with coalition building, oral and written communication, critical thinking, teaching, leadership, policy analysis, policy development, research utilization and technology applications. For example,

- Allow students to provide feedback about the syllabus or an assignment (policy analysis);
- Use a software package in class to pre- and post-test class members opinions about public policy roles for family and consumer sciences (technology applications); and
- Require students to participate in a student organization on campus and volunteer for committee work (leadership, coalition building).

It will be important to the instructor to help make the connection for students with the activities they are doing and the competency they are working toward, particularly at this beginning level. The instructor of such a course should provide not only the experiences with these processes, but also identify for students when they are engaging in the process or using the skill to aid transfer of this learning to other venues. In this initial course the instructor might also want to alert students when a project or paper may be appropriate for their portfolio. A similar approach would be used for attitudes and attributes. The instructor would call to students' attention various opportunities for developing circumstance acuity, common sense, confidence, entrepreneurial thinking and ethical conduct. The class plan should include individual conferences with the instructor during the course and a debriefing conference at the end of the semester with each student. These conferences will include portfolio review and a student self-assessment and instructor assessment of progress toward attaining competencies. This may be viewed as time-intensive work, and it is, but it will establish the necessary foundation for future learning and success in public policy involvement.

CONCLUSION

In speeches spanning the last decade, two distinguished scholars, Kellett (1994) and Vickers (1984), provided direction for the human sciences. Their message: Contributions which can have the greatest impact on families and the society in which they live will come from human scientists who know how to effect change in the public policy arena. This capacity for successful engagement in public policy formation requires the dedicated efforts of a profession to educate its neophytes. The development of prudent curriculum for human sciences undergraduates can have lasting effects on the lives of these young professionals and the families they choose to serve.

NOTES

1. Terms such as family and consumer sciences, home economics, human sciences, human development and applied development science are used interchangeably throughout this chapter.

2. Terms such as public policy involvement, political activity, public policy engagement and public policy development are used interchangeably in this chapter.

REFERENCES

Ambrose, D. (1995). *Leadership: The journey inward.* Dubuque, IA: Kendall/Hunt Publishing Company.

Anderson, C. L. & Miles C. S. (1990). Policy education: Making a difference in the public arena. *Journal of Home Economics, 82,* 7-11.

Andrews, F. C., Mitstifer, D. I., Rehm, M. & Vaughn, G. G. (1995). *Leadership: Reflective human action.* East Lansing, MI: Kappa Omicron Nu.

Andrews, F. E. & Clark, V. L. (1996). Guest editor's message. *Kappa Omicron Nu Forum, 9,* 2-3.

Baldwin, E. E. (1991). The home economics movement: A "new" integrative paradigm. *Journal of Home Economics, 83,* 42-48.

Brown, M. & Paolucci, B. (1979). *Home economics: A definition.* Washington, DC: American Home Economics Association.

Cummings, P. R. (1982). *Home economists and political participation.* Unpublished doctoral dissertation, Oklahoma State University, Stillwater.

Cummings, P. R. & Hirschlein, B. (1984). Shaping the future through political participation. *Journal of Home Economics, 76,* 46-47.

Delli Carpini, M. X. & Keeter, S. (1996). *What Americans know about politics and why it matters.* New Haven, CT: Yale University Press.

Fine, M. A. (1992). Families in the United States: Their current status and future prospects. *Family Relations, 41,* 430-435.

Hammond, K. R. (1996). *Human judgment and social policy.* New York: Oxford University Press.

Jenson, G. O. & Warstadt, T. (1990). *A ranking of critical issues facing American families.* Logan: Utah State University Cooperative Extension Service. (EC No. 435b).

Kellett, C. (1994). Family diversity and difference: A challenge for change. *Journal of Family and Consumer Sciences, 86* (3), 3-11.

Kettl, K., Ingraham, P. W., Sanders, R. P. & Horner, C. (1996). *Civil service reform.* Washington, D.C.: Brookings Institution Press

Laab, J. J. (1994). Women at McDonnell Douglas get political. *Personnel Journal, 43,* 22-29.

Lappé, F. M. & DuBois, P. M. (1994). *The quickening of America.* San Francisco: Jossey-Bass, Inc.

Ley, C. J. (1980). Politically active home economists: Their socialization to politics. *Journal of Vocational Education Research, 5*(3), 29-45.

Ley, C. J. (1982). The key to participation. *J.C. Penney Forum, 11,* 28-31.

Lynn, L. E. (1996). *Public management as art, science and profession.* Chatham, NJ: Chatham House.

Mathews, D. (1994). *Politics for people.* Urbana, IL: University of Illinois.

Meszaros, P. S. & Cummings, P. (1983). Roots in public policy formation. *Journal of Home Economics, 75,* 34-37.

Neruda, G. S. (1979). *A survey of the extent of involvement of professional home economists in public affairs activities.* Unpublished doctoral dissertation, University of Maryland.

Osborne D. & Gaebler, T. (1992). *Reinventing America: How the entrepreneurial spirit is transforming the public sector.* New York: Penguin Books.

Perot, R. & Simon, P. (1996). *The dollar crisis.* Arlington, TX: Summit Publishing Group.

Sheehan, K. & Vaughn, G. (1991). *The legislative process: Becoming an effective advocate.* Alexandria, VA: American Home Economics Association.

Shor, I. (1992). *Empowering education: Critical teaching for social change.* Chicago, IL: The University of Chicago Press.

Skinner, D. A. & Anderson, E. (1993). *Teaching family policy: A handbook of course syllabi, teaching strategies and resources.* Minneapolis, MN: National Council on Family Relations.

Terry, R. W. (1993). *Authentic leadership: Courage in action.* San Francisco: Jossey-Bass.

Theobald, R. (1992). *Turning the century: Personal and organizational strategies for your changed world.* Indianapolis, IN: Knowledge Systems.

Thompson, T. (1996). *Power to the people.* New York: Harper Collins.

Tripple, P. A. (1990). Socialization of students for advocacy roles. *Journal of Home Economics, 82,* 25-27.

Vickers, C. A. (1985). Effective public policy: A question of attitude. *Journal of Home Economics, 77,* 49-53.

Wisensale, S. K. (1992). Toward the 21st century: Family change and public policy. *Family Relations, 41*, 417-422.
Zimmerman, S. L. (1992). Family trends; What implications for family policy? *Family Relations, 41*, 423-429.

Scholarship Reconsidered: A Functional Core for Graduate Curricula

Karen E. Craig and Joan M. Laughlin,
University of Nebraska

Higher education is involved in self-examination relative to its effectiveness in contemporary society. Criticisms from stakeholders—citizens, legislators, governing boards, students and alumni—feed the dialogue about the relevance of the role and mission of higher education in an era of accountability and decreasing resources. As Lynton and Elman (1987) indicated, new priorities must be established because "the nature and importance of knowledge in modern society are changing both quantitatively and qualitatively" (p. 1). Knowledge must be synthesized to be useful. This is as true for the student in the classroom as it is for state and federal legislators, the commissioners in communities, or citizens. While relationships to students and professional societies may have been priority audiences for faculty, the issues present in contemporary society make it essential that faculty in higher education facilitate the use of science and the knowledge base for decision-making in all aspects of society. Priorities for faculty must include responsibility for synthesis of the knowledge base as a means of creating better policy and improving programs. Several factors in higher education that have precluded effective use of the knowledge base in solving societal problems are described below. This is particularly true for problems in human services.

1. *Transfer of Knowledge to Problem Solution.* It is interesting to note that the knowledge base in physical sciences (and engineering) has connected with technology transfer by developing technology or research parks in communities to help in the dissemination and adoption of best practices. This strategy has facilitated the movement of concepts, research output, from development to implementation/adoption in significantly shorter periods of time.
2. *Limited Synthesis and Integration of Knowledge.* Higher education has not emphasized synthesis and integration of knowledge for undergraduate and graduate students. It has fallen victim to the concept of efficiency and mass production as approaches to productivity in society. Emphasis on knowledge and content without concurrent emphasis on building connections with context and factors in complex social issues, may do more harm than good.
3. *Limited Connections of Specializations.* Specialization as it relates to consumers, citizens or clientele has not facilitated the holistic perspective essential to effective solutions of problems in development and delivery of human services. As an example, the Board on Human Sciences sponsored a Welfare Reform Meeting in November of 1996. At that meeting scientists in family life, family economics and child development discovered other disciplines that were interested in the same problems of poverty as they effect the well-being of the family and its members.

4. *Limited Connections among Scholarly Functions.* Lynton and Elman (1987) suggest that teaching, co-curricular, and other professional activities in contemporary higher education must relate theory to practice, basic research to its applications, and acquisition of knowledge to its use. Involvement of faculty and students in external applications of knowledge through policy analysis, technical assistance and extension activities, and broader constructs for scholarly work naturally create a new quest for the use of knowledge by students. Technical competency in a specialized subject matter is necessary, but not sufficient.

In 1990, Boyer created a profound impression on the academy when he asked that scholarship be "reconsidered" for faculty roles. The need to broaden scholarship beyond the generation and dissemination of knowledge was reaffirmed. In a retrospective on American higher education, Boyer's first chapter (1990) characterizes three distinct and overlapping eras/phases in the evolution of contemporary higher education. The first era, the British view of college life, focused on the building of character and preparation of new generations for civic and religious leadership. Throughout the 1800s, higher education continued to evolve another role: service. But it was the end of the 19th century before the third dimension of the role of higher education, research, became a common expectation for higher education. The emphasis on research and graduate education, a relative latecomer to American higher education, has resulted in specialized knowledge geared toward the right answer or fact, with little emphasis on the role of science as a change agent in reducing problems in society.

While faculty saw research with its related publications as the most important dimension of productivity at mid-century, the seeds for changing expectations for universities were planted by a President's Commission on Higher Education in 1947 (Boyer, 1987). The report indicated that higher education must be a means of helping every citizen achieve as much as his or her capacities allow. The shift from elite to mass participation in higher education had begun! Concurrent with the move to mass participation in higher education was a shift in priorities within higher education in which scholarly activities, narrowly defined as research, emerged as the priority for faculty productivity (Lynton & Elman, 1987).

As higher education enters the twenty-first century, two- and four-year degrees have become entitlements. Concurrently, structural shifts in employment, corporate efforts at efficiency, and community needs for revitalization have demanded that higher education assume a greater role in economic development. The next leadership role for higher education as a change agent in society is to provide a source of professionals and/or consultative service providers who assist in the design and implementation of human services programs.

THE CONTEXT OF PROFESSIONAL EDUCATION

Graduate and professional education have been influenced over the years by the expectations of faculty—expectations that reflect the philosophical emphases of the era(s) in which they were educated and that include values, priorities, and ways of defining excellence (Bok, 1986). Faculty often replicate their experience in graduate school as they guide graduate students through curricular, scholarly, and co-curricular experiences. When experiences emphasized research as the scholarly role in higher education, research became the core emphasis in graduate education. Faculty with positive teaching assistant experiences advocated teaching assistantships as important educational experiences in graduate education. Because few faculty had intensive public policy experiences prior to, or in their graduate education experiences, faculty have not advocated for development of a scholarship of integration and application of science to solve problems in society.

While home economics leaders in the 1960s discussed the importance of public policy (Bivens, et al., 1979), there were few who advocated the importance of professional leadership in the design and development of policy as an academic scholarly activity. That probably characterizes the consensus among most professional associations. When policy was included, the efforts were more likely to be directed toward understanding the impact of policy on the clientele to be served and not on the design of good public policy. Another policy role was to write letters advocating for or against a bill, but little effort was directed to development or modification of public programs and policies.

Other professional programs, such as medicine, law and business which require very precise skills for effective practice of professional roles, have experienced the same tension between science, theory, and the development of practical, utilitarian skills essential to effective professional practice. In contrast, programs in the arts and sciences have been designed to develop academics. Both medicine and law experience tension in concurrently developing professional expertise of both the subject matter and application of the subject matter. It is to be expected that graduate education in applied programs will experience the same tension. Students and faculty perceive moral dilemmas and social responsibility as secondary to the need to master the knowledge and skills of the profession (Bok, 1986). Neither students nor faculty have held in high esteem the integration of knowledge to address the policy issues in society.

Professional education is largely a result of the interplay of several constituencies, intellectual factors, experiences, and attitudes of the faculty. In periods of external change, the tendency is to continue to do things the way they have been done. Examination of past practices and needs for the society is not a positive alternative for faculty in a changing higher education environment.

FORMAT FOR SCHOLARSHIP SERVING PUBLIC POLICY

Boyer (1990) in *Scholarship Reconsidered* provides a broad construct for excellence in contemporary faculty roles. His framework also provides a model for conceptualizing graduate education for persons interested in public policy advocacy, development and implementation. Boyer's four concepts—discovery, integration, application, and teaching—provide an interesting strategy for design of graduate professional education. Applying the concepts of the new scholarship to graduate education could assure educational experiences for students which build professional competency with science, the knowledge base, as well as skills for the integration and application of that knowledge in developing solutions to real problems in society.

Discovery. The basis of graduate education must continue to include research competencies. Within a dynamic society, the knowledge base continues to change and evolve in response to the social and economic environment. Kerlinger (1986) describes the aim of science as theory development. Understanding the current state of the human condition is essential to solving problems.

While emphasis on the research component may appear to have been overemphasized, a strong research base is part of the core education essential to designing policies and programs that alleviate societal problems. Building programs on science, the knowledge base, is the only way to assure a greater chance of success for the future. Science must reflect the complete research cycle. See Figure 3.1 for a conceptualization of the research cycle as a process where theory is tested through models and concepts which provide explanations and change practice and policy (Laughlin, 1995).

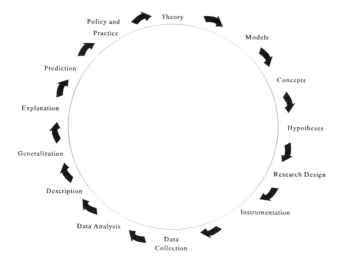

Figure 3.1 Model of Research Cycle.

As can be seen in the model, the intervening parts of the model are hypotheses, design, instrumentation, data collection, analysis and description of results, generalization, explanation and prediction. Laughlin (1995) observes that the full model of research is often short circuited with explanations used as the beginning of the next research cycle without addressing the issues of prediction, policy and practice. Prediction, policy and practice are important in providing additional insight about the theory which then contributes to new research models with new concepts contributing to new explanations and so on.

Integration. Drawing together and bringing insight to bear on original research, integration (Boyer, 1990) is the connection of the small pieces within disciplines and across disciplines. Integration is the interpretation of what has been discovered to provide a larger more comprehensive understanding of the significance of the facts. Integration always involves synthesis of information and often is built on multidisciplinary concepts. It has been a neglected aspect in education and research in recent history. Science, in the process of discovery or research, has reduced every problem to its smallest unit (reductionist perspective) and built a knowledge base on the small segments assuming that the many parts would be additive and result in a more accurate big picture. However, sometimes the results make no sense. Integration is essential if we are to correct these nonsense collections of facts. It builds the connections between facts and disciplines to address the critical issues in society.

Application. This scholarly role focuses on how knowledge can be responsibly applied to consequential problems in society. When theory and practice interact, each renews the other. New intellectual understandings arise from the act of application—medical diagnosis, serving clients, shaping public policy, or working in other settings (Boyer, 1990). This view of scholarly activity, one that both applies and contributes to human knowledge, is particularly needed in a world in which the huge, complex problems require the skills and insights inherent in the academy.

Teaching. As teaching is the highest form of understanding, teaching at its best is transmitting knowledge and transforming and extending it as well. Faculty who involve students in reading, discussions and reflection on the application of knowledge in the teaching/learning environment develop competencies for being advocates or designers of public policy reflecting the research base associated with the problem.

APPLICATION OF THE NEW SCHOLARSHIP MODEL TO PUBLIC POLICY ACTIVITIES

Figure 3.2 identifies specific professional activities as they relate to the analysis and design of public policies and programs. They are categorized by three of Boyer's dimensions of the New Scholarship. Teaching, the fourth concept would incorporate the other three.

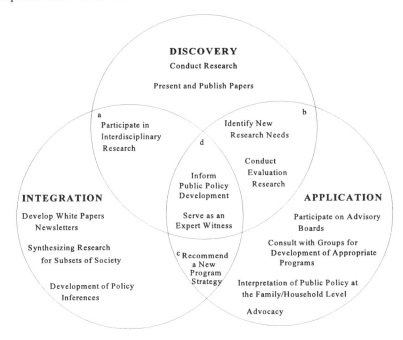

Figure 3.2 Professional Roles in Public Policy.

Effective practice as a policy professional includes analysis, design, and implementation skills—the three aspects of discovery, integration, and application and the intersections between the three.

Intersection a. For example, participation in multidisciplinary or interdisciplinary research requires integration and synthesis skills to create the solutions which reflect multiple disciplines. The multiple perspectives define different research questions that result from a single discipline perspective. The multiple perspectives define different research questions than result from a single discipline perspective.

Intersection b. The connection or overlap between application and discovery involves identification of new research needs (the extension/research connection inherent in the land-grant system). Likewise, program assessment and evaluation research requires application of research skills to programs. Evaluation research is charged with identifying the effectiveness of the program in creating desired changes in behavior or conditions.

Intersection c. Recommendation of a new program strategy requires a synthesis of the impact of current applications as they relate to the problem to be solved and an application of knowledge to other factors in the environment to create solutions. Each new application requires integration of knowledge from different disciplines to address problems in diverse settings.

Intersection d. Serving as an expert witness or helping design policy requires facts and synthesis and integration of those facts from a variety of sources. It culminates in application to develop a solution of a particular problem. As an expert witness, the solution is for one person or a homogeneous group. With policy work, the solution is for a class or group of persons with a common problem.

Each of these roles is important in effectively using the knowledge base to design programs to change the quality of life of citizens. Actions taken without the benefit of these scholarly roles serves neither clientele nor citizens well.

APPLICATION OF THE NEW SCHOLARSHIP TO GRADUATE EDUCATION

Graduate education and training experiences have the capacity to socialize future scholars to the processes of teaching, research, and service. It will not happen unless scholars, faculty and graduate students, are provided the opportunity to study, observe, interpret, interact, experience and work in mentor/teamwork environments which develop attitudes and skills for providing the objective knowledge imperative to development of policies which enhance the human condition (Paulson & Feldman, 1995).

Figure 3.3 provides a series of educational experiences which could be associated with graduate education to develop in students the expertise to be full participants in the development of public programs and policies.

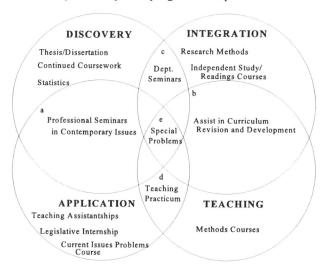

Figure 3.3 Educational Experiences for Graduate Public Policy Education.

As in the professional roles, the application of the concepts of the new scholarship provides a framework for analysis of experiences for graduate students. The circles represent the four dimensions of the new scholarship—discovery, integration, application, and teaching. Activities associated with effective graduate education are identified in each circle as they represent strategies for developing competency for effective participation in public policy. Note that none of the activities is a new activity for graduate education. The activities are simply organized to create specific skills.

The intersections, a through e, represent other existing graduates experiences that can build on the dynamics of the four dimensions of scholarly work.

Intersection a. Participation in professional seminars brings both discovery techniques and application skills to the setting of contemporary issues. These experiences focus on bringing the science, facts from several disciplines, to reflect on particular problems in society and as such, evolve new research theories, models, to build the science.

Intersection b. Assistance with the design, review and revision of classroom activities as they relate to student needs provides an opportunity to build on the dynamics of synthesis and teaching as they occur in the classroom. Curricular change that requires greater student responsibility for learning develops student capacity to reorganize facts in the context of the learning situation.

Intersection c. Department seminars which focus on the methodology and theory associated with research provide the opportunity to develop skills for conceptualizing issues in policy as they relate to integration of various parts of the research or knowledge base. Department seminars which focus on interpretation of the facts from a discipline perspective as building blocks for new theory development build student skills to synthesize and integrate in development of research programs which contribute to new policies.

Intersection d. A teaching practica provides the opportunity to apply concepts in a supervised learning environment. While a teaching assistantship provides similar experience, there is substantial variation in the level of development and supervision associated with teaching assistantships. A teaching practica provides focus and supervision for teaching/learning with a master which builds on synthesis and integration skills of the mentor/supervisor.

Intersection e. Special problems courses provide the opportunity to create alternatives for policy using all four dimensions of the new scholarship. The flexibility here could enhance skills for design of policy in a variety of professional settings, including academic, legislative, program management, and consultative. They may even provide the opportunity to design, deliver, and assess a new policy and/or program.

CONCLUSIONS

Policy is the result of a sense of community and feelings of mutual responsibility for the well-being of the citizens. Graduates of programs conceptualized from the new scholarship model can be effective team members—leaders, participants and consultants in designing public policy which serves the well-being of members of the society and economy.

Application of the concepts of the new scholarship—discovery, integration, application and teaching—to graduate curricula can assure educational experiences which build professional competency with the knowledge base as well as the skills essential for integration and application of that knowledge for analysis, design, and implementation of policies.

REFERENCES

Bivens, G., Fitch, M., Newkirk, G., Paolucci, B., Riggs, E., St. Marie, S., & Vaughn, G. (1979). Home Economics—New Directions II. In Bonnie Rader (Ed.) *Significant writings in home economics: 1911-1979* (pp. 159-162). Peoria, IL: Glencoe Publishing Company.

Bok, D. (1986). *Higher learning.* Cambridge, MA: Harvard University Press.

Boyer, E. L. (1990). *Scholarship reconsidered: Priorities for the professoriate.* Princeton, N.J.: The Carnegie Foundation for the Advancement of Teaching.

Kerlinger, F. N. (1986). *Foundations of behavioral research. Third Edition.* Fort Worth, Texas: Harcourt Brace.

Laughlin, J. (1995). Unpublished materials for HRFS 875, Research Methods.

Lynton, E. A. & Elman, S. E. (1987). *New priorities for the university: Meeting society's needs for applied knowledge and competent individuals.* San Francisco: Jossey-Bass.

Paulson, M. B. & Feldman, K. A. (1995). Toward a reconceptualization of scholarship: a human action system with functional imperatives. *Journal of Higher Education, 66*(6), 615-640.

Creating Communities of Practice for Experiential Learning in Policy Studies
Charles McClintock, *Cornell University*

Educating students for social policy and management roles in the twenty-first century requires attention to a wide range of challenges in higher education. These include integrating classroom and field study, balancing a liberal arts education for breadth and perspective with pre-professional specialization for immediate post-graduate demands, understanding the interplay between scientific and social bases of knowledge, and joining the goals of diversity—from intellectual and moral perspectives to human attributes and social groups—with communal values and commitments. The difficulty of these challenges notwithstanding, it is an exciting time for social policy education given that the significant changes underway in social welfare, health, and education create enormous opportunities to engage students in field study and research (McClintock & Beck, 1998; McClintock & Colosi, 1998).

There is an urgency to think imaginatively about policy education that is grounded in the complexity of current social problems and also assessed by rigorous academic standards. The necessity for new approaches is heightened in light of the sobering statistics regarding economic and social trends and disparities for America's poorest children and families (Bronfenbrenner, McClelland, Wethington, Moen & Ceci, 1996). These include the problems of underemployment and low-income growth, child abuse, out-of-wedlock childbearing, imprisonment of relatively high proportions of ethnic minority populations, and various health-status problems for low-income groups. In order to address these pressing problems, Lerner and Fisher (1994) have defined an applied developmental science framework that provides an intellectual vision for policy education. This perspective emphasizes the need for cross-disciplinary collaboration among scholars, and a contextualized and ecological understanding of human development as it evolves across the life course and interweaves varied physical, biological and social environments.

In a turbulent policy environment, the ties that bind higher education to society can be strengthened through collaboration among academicians, policy makers, front-line human service managers and practitioners, and citizens (McClintock, 1999). These collaborative efforts can be designed to demonstrate the mutual relevance of the scholarship of discovery which emphasizes creation of new knowledge through research, and the scholarship of application with its focus on the integration of theory and practice (Boyer, 1990). Engaging these different groups in educational *communities of practice* can advance the complementary goals of rigorously creating contextualized knowledge about human development, evaluating the effects of public policy in ways that truly inform program development at the local level, and ultimately improving the well-being of individuals, families, and communities. Given the need for educational boundary spanning between campus and community, policy studies curricula that integrate field and classroom learning are critical, and provide the pedagogical component for

Bronfenbrenner's (1979) ecological framework for understanding and improving human development in its various real-world contexts.

CREATING COMMUNITIES OF PRACTICE

The concept of an educational community of practice (Lave & Wenger, 1991)—ongoing reflective interaction among students, faculty, policy and service practitioners, and citizens—is fundamental to both professional and liberal arts perspectives on learning. This kind of situated learning links education to its social context through specific mechanisms such as apprenticeships (Hamilton, 1990), experiential learning (Kolb, 1984), service learning (Jacoby & Associates, 1996), critical discourse (Moore, 1990), and partnerships between academia and community stakeholders (Lerner & Fisher, 1994). Communities of practice are similar to Boyer's (1994) vision of a new American college which would have a mission

> . . . of connecting thought to action and theory to practice. This New American College would organize in cross-disciplinary ways around pressing social issues. Undergraduates would participate in field projects, relating ideas to real life. Classrooms and laboratories would be extended to include health clinics, youth centers, schools and government offices. Faculty members would build partnerships with practitioners who would, in turn, come to campus as lecturers and student advisors. (p. A-48)

Proposals such as this which emphasize an active interplay between field and campus environments often are caught in an academic cross-fire over *rigor versus relevance*. One position holds that internships and field research projects provide the truest test of knowledge through application in the "messy" real world, whereas the more traditional view disputes the intellectual value of such experiences while granting their potential role in students' personal growth and professional training (Moore, 1990). This debate tends to center in the social sciences because field study, or its parent pedagogy experiential learning, are not as well accepted as in the arts and natural sciences where studio and laboratory work are considered essential to learning. Regardless of its intellectual status, a key issue for any experiential pedagogy, especially when applied to the changing and fast-paced world of policy and management, is to specify and evaluate the knowledge and learning goals in ways that are comparable in rigor to assessing classroom education.

Schön (1983, 1987) demonstrated that the "rigor versus relevance" dichotomy has a long tradition manifest in the academy's attitude toward professionally oriented education, but that rigor is miscast as residing only in basic scientific knowledge which in turn rests on a theory of knowledge that is incomplete. In his view, the traditional positivist orientation, in which knowledge derived and validated from research is then passed on to the practitioner to apply, has led to misplaced confidence in technocratic approaches as illustrated in social and political crises such as the Vietnam War.

Taking schooling as an example, others have argued that the limited impact of educational research on teaching and learning is due in part to an overemphasis on control of variables and a disregard for practitioner knowledge, when it is in fact complex multivariate contexts and professional discretion that are key to implementing knowledge in the classroom (Brown, et al., 1989; Kennedy, 1997). In this view, the goal is not to control or eliminate confounding factors, but to accommodate them by involving professionals, clients and citizens in field research along with researchers and students in the development, evaluation and implementation of policy. In short, viewing knowledge as a unidirectional flow from laboratory to field overlooks the fact that scientific knowledge has a socially constructed and enacted component by which its meaning and influence on human affairs is determined through culture, social interaction, reflection and negotiation.

Schön (1983) maintains that the social and policy problems confronted by professionals—doctors, designers, engineers, human service practitioners, administrators, lawyers—require a new kind of discovery and reflection emphasizing the tacit knowledge[1] that resides in the best examples of artistry and wisdom in professional practice. His emphasis on the "epistemology of practice" is summarized in the vision of a "reflective practitioner" who seeks effectiveness in settings that typically contain: 1) uncertainty about problem definition and intervention impact, 2) uniqueness of problem-solving situations, and 3) value conflict that is not resolvable through technical means alone. In this environment, the most effective practitioners draw upon research and experience-based knowledge that is both general and case specific, causal and moral, and applied in strategic ways that transcend barriers in practice which often appear intractable (Shulman, 1986).

This vision of reflective practice and the interplay between tacit and research-based knowledge need not be driven solely by a concern with professional education. Anderson (1993), in writing about the need to invigorate liberal arts education, uses the term "practical reason" in a way comparable to Schön's concept of the reflective practitioner. He links general learning from the liberal arts curriculum to its societal value through a set of basic intellectual habits and values that focuses on preparing "people to think, plan, judge, empathize, wonder, hypothesize, criticize, test, invent and imagine" (Anderson, 1993, p. 3).

These student attributes represent the ideals of a community of practice in policy studies, or for that matter, any field. Hence, experiential teaching and learning that combine explicit and tacit knowledge is more than just applying theory to practice and then enumerating situation-specific rules and procedures. It requires attention to how knowledge is created, tested and transformed through improvisation, insight and interplay between conceptual and action-based learning. Teaching students generalizable knowledge from the often disconnected particulars of subject matter, professional practice and everyday experience is a core component of both liberal arts and professional education (McClintock, 1990a).

Schön's work (1983), which itself is grounded in Dewey's (1986) philosophical pragmatism and the significance of practical inquiry, offers a provocative treatment of experiential learning that combines rigor and relevance through micro-experimentation and master class formats to make explicit the tacit knowledge of professional expertise. At the same time, however, there is a continued need for emphasis on assessing student learning from such efforts, since much of the literature on experiential learning at the undergraduate level is less specific on intellectual growth, emphasizing instead other important benefits such as students' professional preparation, personal growth or service to the community that often result from internships, apprenticeships, and other field study projects.

How might knowledge and learning goals based in communities of practice be operationally defined for policy education programs based in developmental science? The beginnings of an answer to this question can be created in three ways: 1) articulating a pedagogical framework for field study that integrates the tacit knowledge of policy and management professionals with research-based knowledge, 2) illustrating potential content of an undergraduate curriculum in policy analysis and management, and 3) outlining a research and curriculum development agenda around tacit knowledge that will help faculty rigorously assess integrated field and classroom learning. The final point is especially important if field study is to be widely implemented, since specifying subject matter content will help elevate the intellectual value of experiential knowledge for faculty by clarifying its effect on student learning (Stanton & Giles, 1989).

FIELD STUDY PEDAGOGY IN SOCIAL POLICY PROGRAMS

Experiential learning covers a broad range of activities from in-class exercises such as case analysis, role playing, and computer simulation, to the lab, studio and practicum, and finally to field study situations such as internships, externships and field research.   Learning from field study is challenging because students are expected to integrate conceptual and research-based knowledge with skilled activity and problem solving in settings which are heavily influenced by practitioners' tacit knowledge reflecting a mixture of cultural, social and professional expertise. Also, because field study is often structured around work in a specific internship or research project, it represents a special challenge for the teacher to help students maintain a focus on and a demonstration of their intellectual development around general concepts and principles. For all these reasons, too, it is in field study settings that faculty can be most challenged intellectually as teacher-scholars, since their own training may have placed more emphasis on the formal theories and methods of their disciplines and less on their application in policy and practitioner settings.   Hence, faculty development in experiential learning, and field study in particular, is critical to the success of this pedagogy.

Despite these challenges, there are sound pedagogical grounds for investing in field study that integrates conceptual knowledge within a social and problem-solving context, starting with conceptions of human intelligence and learning. For example, Sternberg's (1985) triarchic theory of intelligence goes beyond the abstract cognitive skills traditionally measured by IQ to distinguish three subsystems—cognitive, experiential and contextual—each of which accounts for critical aspects of intellectual performance.   The cognitive or componential subsystem represents the mechanisms by which knowledge is acquired and conceptually structured.   The experiential subsystem represents the capacity for creativity and skilled performance in moving from familiar to novel tasks and settings, and the contextual subsystem specifies the capacity to adapt to, select, and shape the sociocultural environment.

A compatible approach to the analysis of intelligence is provided by Gardner (1993) whose theory proffers seven primary forms of intelligence that individuals possess in varying degrees—linguistic, musical, logical-mathematical, spatial, body-kinesthetic, intrapersonal (e.g., insight, metacognition), and interpersonal (e.g., social skills). Gardner's system has direct implications for field study in terms of providing varied learning experiences and modes of assessment that will allow students' distinct profiles of competence to flourish.

Kolb's (1984) model of experiential learning provides an application of this perspective with his cyclical process in which students have concrete experience (CE), engage in reflective observation on it (RO), develop abstract conceptualizations (AC) from this reflection on action, pursue active experimentation (AE) to test this abstracted knowledge, and begin the cycle over with new experience that builds off the results of experimentation. Kolb relates these phases of learning to two underlying dimensions—CE or RO which is about how directly one grasps experience and AC or AE emphasizing how abstractly one analyzes or transforms experience—which lead to his companion concept of individual learning styles. For example, using Kolb's Learning Styles Inventory, students can be classified as having one of four distinctive perceptual and cognitive approaches: divergent (CE/RO), assimilative (AC/RO), convergent (AC/AE) and accommodative CE/AE). The point of this example, regardless of its specific validity, is to emphasize that field pedagogy and assessment should reflect different learning phases and possibly preferred learner styles, and that it will be enriched by including complementary contributions from a diverse team of students, faculty and various field participants.

If intelligence is multifaceted in ways such as those described by Sternberg (1985) and Gardner (1993), including both its practical/situational and abstract forms, and learning phases and styles vary in their instructional requirements according to Kolb, how can field study be used to enhance education in policy and management settings? The ideas of situated learning (Brown, Collins & Duguid, 1989) and communities of practice (Lave & Wenger, 1991) provide part of the answer. Situated learning is a function of the activity, context and culture in which it occurs which stands in contrast with most classroom learning that emphasizes abstract and decontextualized knowledge. In situated learning, students absorb the reasons for, and meanings of, action in a particular professional context, and it is the job of their mentors to help them reflect on this information in critical ways. Social interaction is a key component of situated learning in the sense that learners become involved in communities of practice which emphasize skilled activities, professional and cultural beliefs and values, and to a lesser extent general concepts. This highly heterogeneous teaching and learning environment provides opportunities for students to find perspectives, modalities of learning and forms for expression of knowledge that draw on the strengths of their backgrounds and learning styles. The task of the faculty member or field mentor is made correspondingly more complex, however, both in structuring learning opportunities and evaluating student performance (McClintock & Beck, 1998).

Applying situated learning and communities of practice to educating undergraduates in policy studies requires learning in an adult world of professional practice, and provides a foundation for identifying and assessing tacit knowledge. Similar to theories of adult learning (e.g., Knowles, 1984) which emphasize the value of experiential and problem-solving approaches, field study that is situated in professional contexts can enhance the motivation to learn by clarifying the immediate value and application of the knowledge. In the social policy arena, this value would center on those individuals, communities, and institutions that are the intended beneficiaries of human sciences.

Similarly, service-learning (Jacoby & Associates, 1996)—a term that has come to express a set of values toward field study of service to others, individual and community empowerment, and reciprocal control and learning between those being served and the learners—becomes an important part of the pedagogy of field study in social policy. The service-learning approach to field study in policy education not only has sound pedagogical bases in research on cognition and learning, but also is integral to a wide range of broader social policy efforts emphasizing communitarian thinking (Etzioni, 1995), volunteer action and the not-for-profit community agency sector (Rifkin, 1995), and the role of higher education in promoting civic life (Gamson, 1997). The range of resources and activities linking the campus to the community has grown rapidly over the past decade (e.g., Sirianni & Friedland, 1997), and hearkens to much earlier conceptions of education and community such as Dewey's laboratory school and Tocqueville's observations of voluntary groups. These linkages between field study and community become even more important in an era of devolution of social policy and programs from federal to state and local levels.

Notwithstanding these service-oriented and situation-specific pedagogical features of field study, learning also requires the refinement of conceptual structures within which knowledge is organized. Reflecting on field and classroom knowledge together relies heavily on an ability to conceptualize situations from a variety of perspectives and to integrate setting-specific and abstract learning (Hutchings & Wutzdorff, 1988).

The task of integrating the concrete knowledge from field study with more abstract knowledge can be approached using concept mapping. Novak and Gowin (1984) describe concept maps and the process for developing and using them to assess student learning. In their approach to teaching and learning with concept maps, students are taught how to construct conceptual frameworks for organizing and generalizing knowledge, whether derived from the classroom or field experience, by identifying important concepts, specifying their interrelationships, and linking them to specified observable information. These concept map frameworks are richer and more malleable than content overviews and summaries which simply emphasize key ideas without interconnections and varying levels of abstraction among them.

Most importantly, in Novak and Gowin's analysis, knowledge structures built around concept maps lead to more effective and lasting learning by emphasizing the meaning of ideas through their lateral and hierarchical relationships and linkages with testable evidence. In addition, concept maps can be used as a bridge between learning new content and the student's existing cognitive schema by highlighting the psychological and social context of the learner in constructing knowledge. Concept maps of the same subject matter can look very different depending on the student's prior knowledge and experience, the social context for applying the map, and the content being emphasized by the teacher. Iterative concept maps also provide a chronology of learning as concepts and relationships among them are added and refined, whether based on experiential or classroom learning processes.

An example of a concept map is shown in Figure 4.1 which was used for a program evaluation field research project on hospice services (McClintock, 1990b). The map represented a "community of practice" model for field study in that it was developed iteratively by students and faculty from theoretical and policy literature, input from key professionals in a statewide hospice support organization, individual and focus group interviews with agency administrators, service delivery staff, volunteers and caregivers of deceased clients. In this way, it linked research-based concepts—systems theory in the study of organizations, medical and social psychological aspects of terminal illness, and hospice services—with practitioner and client knowledge of key hospice care elements into a program theory of hospice care causal effects and implementation mechanisms.

The concept map organizes hospice care into hierarchically related concepts including the guiding assumptions (top row of concepts), service components or care activities (middle three rows of concepts), and the causal processes and evidence by which hospice is expected to benefit clients (bottom row of concepts). It served three major purposes in the field study course: 1) as an overview of the domain of inquiry and guide for program evaluation data gathering on various philosophical and programmatic elements of hospice care; 2) as a teaching and learning guide for integrating the breadth of conceptual and practitioner knowledge that went into formulating its components; and 3) as a focal point for examining varying interpretations of concepts (e.g., among health practitioners and families regarding the use of strong medication for symptom and pain management).

Several diverse aspects of field study pedagogy have thus far been identified—emerging concepts of intelligence, situated learning and communities of practice, adult and service learning, campus-community partnerships related to social issues such as volunteerism and welfare reform, and the use of concept maps as a tool for integrating knowledge from the classroom and the field. One way of summarizing these pedagogical underpinnings of field study in social policy programs, albeit a possibly counterintuitive one, is the term "theorizing." Though it may sound abstract, theorizing is a highly practical skill in a world that is increasingly complex, heterogeneous, and democratic. As the social psychologist Kurt Lewin puts it, "there's nothing so practical as a good theory," referring to the value of examining diverse real-world problems with common underlying concepts. Teaching students to theorize is a common thread that can tie together more effectively the worlds of liberal arts and professional education, basic and applied research, and the teaching and research functions of faculty (McClintock, 1990a).

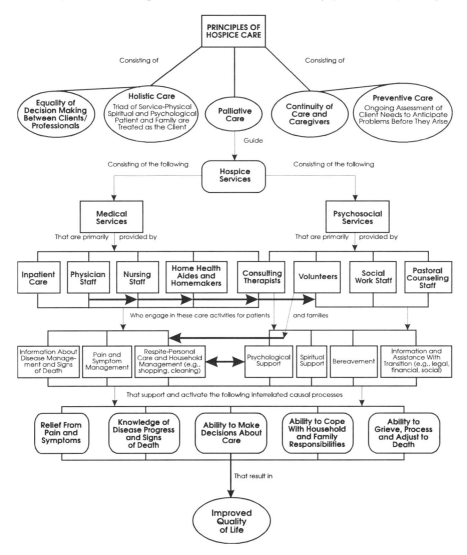

Figure 4.1 A Concept Map of the Program Theory for Hospice Services.

The best scientific theories are those that explain observations parsimoniously and predict future events, but the process of theorizing is not like that. It can be messy, inspired, clumsy, rigorous, uncertain, systematic, and even embarrassing at times. Teaching others how to theorize requires that they account for specific and disparate facts by formulating abstract conceptual frameworks with hypotheses that can be examined empirically. However, it also means transforming concepts into new frameworks by using metaphor, analogy, and examples that don't fit the rule.

Thus, theorizing is a process that moves back and forth between the abstract and the observable, revises what was taken for granted, includes what was overlooked, reframes with analogy, complicates with unexpected findings, and simplifies with new interpretations.

In these ways, theorizing describes a goal for linking the social and situated aspects of field study with the conceptual and intellectual aspects of learning. Teaching students to think theoretically, whether in the laboratory, classroom, neighborhood or workplace, is an underlying educational goal that gives them the capacity to integrate diverse perspectives and be critical of their own observation, inference and conceptual processes. When students learn generalizable knowledge from the interplay of classroom and field settings, they build skills that will help them cope with important dimensions of social policy and practice (e.g., uncertainty, uniqueness and value conflict), that as noted earlier are characteristic of many settings where professionals are challenged to show creativity and wisdom (Schön, 1983).

CURRICULAR CONTENT FOR SOCIAL POLICY PROGRAMS

A comprehensive description of social policy curricular content is not feasible in this paper, but as noted above, linking this content to field study and assessing the degree to which it has been *learned and enriched* from that activity often is the Achilles heel of experiential pedagogy. Hence, several critical aspects of social policy and management content will be described as foci for learning that integrate field and classroom study.

In a recent round of strategic planning at Cornell University, the College of Human Ecology outlined goals for undergraduate education that summarize several key components of curriculum relevant to social policy as well as other academic programs (McClintock, 1994).

> The college will encourage innovative teaching and learning in a context of applied knowledge that reinforces the college's focus on problem-solving for diverse human needs. The undergraduate curriculum will provide a balance between general education and specialization. Students will become reflective professionals who integrate knowledge with interaction skills to improve human welfare. . . . Undergraduate learning should reflect a balance between the intellectual depth required for specific majors and college-wide learning goals for all students. College-wide educational goals should emphasize:
> • *Cognitive skills* (for example, skills for critical thinking and quantitative literacy, visual literacy and analysis, the capacity for knowledge creation, creative problem-solving, reflection on professional practice);
> • *Interpersonal skills* (such as leadership and innovation, ability for teamwork and cooperation, oral and written communication); and
> • *Interdependence and social responsibility* (for example, a sense of community, interdependence and service, understanding and appreciation of diversity and how concepts of human difference are created, the ability to manage a diverse and

changing social, technological and material environment). (p. 12-13)

The three categories of educational accomplishment—intellectual, interpersonal, and interdependence/social responsibility—provide a general framework within which the appraisal of field instruction could begin. Some of the specific educational content within each category is oriented toward policy process knowledge (e.g., leadership, reflection on professional practice), while other parts emphasize policy content (e.g., human diversity, quantitative literacy). Although both are necessary in policy studies and should serve as foci for enhancing learning through field study, the remaining comments will focus primarily on policy content issues since advancing the status of field study among the professoriate requires greater emphasis on subject matter to be learned than typically has been the case with this form of teaching.

Human Diversity

Educating students about human diversity—from ethnicity and gender to political beliefs and moral values—and how concepts of diversity are socially constructed is one critical aspect of social policy programs that has direct relevance for student experience (McClintock & Beck, 1998). For example, living arrangements and social relations among students on college campuses reflect an unresolved struggle between the equally valid needs for forced integration and for voluntary segregation among different racial and ethnic groups. Society has yet to forge a political consensus that embraces the need for both processes, and there still is enormous division over the extent to which historical patterns of discrimination should constitute an explicit political agenda. Public backlash against perceived entitlements to protection and redress creates a palpable tension in public discourse as well as in the classroom.

This tension can inhibit learning simply through avoidance or a one-sided presentation of such policy-related issues as political ideology, ethnicity, racism and policy debates on family and social welfare programs.

University education, and especially social policy studies, should provide students with educational opportunities to experience diversity and to understand historical and contemporary forces that influence how concepts of human difference are created and maintained. This goal can best be furthered by insuring that diversity, in terms of ideas, values, personal characteristics, and culture, is well represented among students and faculty (Bensimon & Soto, 1997). Further, given the rarefied atmosphere of the college campus, it is important to place students in work and social settings where human differences are both stark and subtle, and require them to study, discuss and reflect on the meaning of these experiences. Students also need to experience the conditions that bridge difference and create unity. The experiential component to this kind of teaching is also crucial, because it is easy to become enmeshed in the "culture wars" rhetoric regarding diversity and multicultural issues, while losing sight of common purposes.

Other Policy Curricular Content

The creation of a new academic department in Cornell's College of Human Ecology, the Department of Policy Analysis and Management (PAM), offers another way to illustrate policy studies curricular content that could be taught through field study. The academic plan for PAM specifies a core curriculum and concentrations in health, family/social welfare, and consumer policy and management subject matter that have particular relevance for applied developmental and social sciences (McClintock, 1996). The vision of the new department links policy analysis with program implementation through inclusion of the quantitative modeling approach with management and service delivery content including qualitative methods. This integration of two approaches to policy that are often separate—analysis and implementation—is consistent with views on the future of public policy and management programs based on surveying the field of American institutions (Averch & Dluhy, 1992).

Despite a wide range of academic backgrounds among the faculty in PAM, a decision was made by the faculty and college administration to emphasize economics as a base discipline in the curriculum. This choice rested on the recognition of the significance of economic concepts (e.g., markets, incentives, cost analysis, public finance) to social policy questions along with the more integrated conceptual approach within economics in comparison with other social sciences. At the same time, however, management and related processes of program planning, service delivery and program evaluation, were deemed critical to undergraduate learning in this new department. Cross-cutting all these educational components, was the idea of "critical perspectives" on policy which highlight the social, cultural and political dimensions of how policies are framed and experienced.

As stated in the steering committee report (McClintock, 1996), PAM's teaching mission is to prepare students *as leaders in policy analysis and management in the non-profit, profit and public sectors.* It is expected that undergraduates, in addition to pursuing post-graduate study, will work in government, business, and non-profit organizations in such careers as policy analysts, health and human service providers and managers, consumer advocate and finance specialists, and marketing researchers. More specific learning objectives include:

- Knowledge of public policy issues and programs in the areas of family, welfare, health, consumer and human services as they are affected by government, business and community forces;
- The ability to conceptualize and analyze policy and management issues using models and techniques from the social sciences;
- Insight into cultural diversity and how to work effectively with and deliver services to individuals and families from diverse backgrounds;
- An understanding of program planning, evaluation and management strategies in a variety of human service and corporate settings;
- Knowledge about government institutions and political behavior, and an understanding of how to create and change policies in a political environment;
- The ability to present ideas effectively through written, oral and visual communication; and
- Hands-on experience in analyzing real-world policy and management issues and in developing strategies and systems for addressing them.

In addition to a three-course research methods and statistics core, the curriculum consists of the following courses:

> *Critical Perspectives on Public Policy Issues* introduces students to the critical analysis of contemporary and continuing policy issues from multiple perspectives.

> *Introduction to Policy Analysis* addresses fundamental concepts of policy analysis and public sector functioning.

Introduction to Management of Service Organizations builds a foundation in leadership, management and implementation skills relevant to public, non-profit and private sector settings.

Intermediate Microeconomics for Policy Analysis presents economic and decision theory paradigms to the analysis of social programs in the public and private sectors.

Applied Public Finance provides an overview of the public sector of the U.S. economy, major categories of public expenditures, and the methods to finance these expenditures.

As can be seen from Figure 4.2 (McClintock, 1996), field study can pertain to any of these core courses as well as courses in particular policy and practice concentrations that students develop.

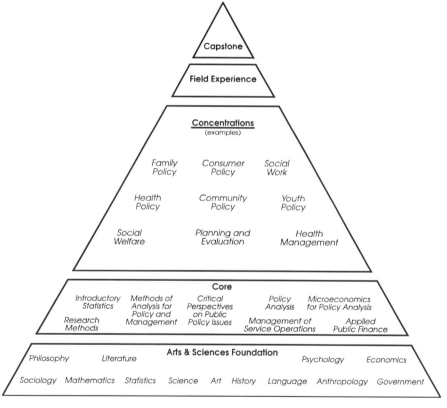

Figure 4.2 Undergraduate Policy and Management Curriculum.

The range of policy and management issues that could be explored through field study and internships in this curriculum is quite wide and could apply to many of the concerns identified in applied developmental science as described by Lerner and Fisher (1994). Significantly, the PAM faculty endorsed an honors program in

44

Social Change, Public Policy, and Community Collaborations: Training
Human Development Professionals for the Twenty-First Century

experiential learning parallel to research honors, in which students emphasize first-hand exposure to professional practices in human service policy analysis and management. A few examples are drawn from the topic of welfare reform because the breadth of current change in this policy area is so central to applied developmental science. Each issue offers an opportunity to create a community of practice through field work in which research-based knowledge is intermixed with knowledge from practitioners, clients and communities.

Workforce attachment. Moving individuals from public assistance to work is the centerpiece of welfare policy change. Students can assess the barriers to long-term employment, including economic, social and psychological issues, and evaluate the effectiveness of training programs relative to client needs. School-to-work apprenticeship programs offer opportunities to involve students in partnerships with educators and employers to seek long-term solutions to meaningful youth and young adult employment based on policy approaches from other countries. Value perspectives on the role of government, the private sector and individual responsibility offer a rich array of inquiry for field study in this area.

Child care. Many assistance recipients are single parents who need reliable, flexible, and affordable child care that leaves them secure enough to pursue employment with changing shifts and transportation barriers that make it difficult to reach children during work hours. In addition, assistance recipients can satisfy work requirements by providing child care. Students could explore how to identify appropriate caregivers and the skills needed for effective care, forecast supply and demand, as well as compare the benefits to be expected from various types of center-based and family-based care models. From an economic perspective, students might study the cost-benefit tradeoffs of local community investment in childcare as a means to facilitate moving from public assistance to employment.

Teenage pregnancy and non-marital births. New federal and state legislation contains incentives, time limits and restrictions to reduce teenage pregnancy. Students could explore the underlying social and behavioral factors that cause these problems and evaluate the extent to which the policy incentives are having the intended effects. Related policy issues that could serve as opportunities for internships or field research include enforcing new paternity determination and child support enforcement policies, and assessing their effects on parental participation in children's lives.

Services for children and families. Students can learn about the skills needed by a wide range of human service professionals—home visitors, social service case managers, community health workers, teachers aides—in a policy environment that emphasizes employment, family strengths, prevention, community-based accessible services, service coordination, integration and accountability. The design and evaluation of training programs for professionals and paraprofessionals also offer opportunities for student involvement.

Human service planning and evaluation. Block grants and reduced funding formulas will create incentives and needs for service coordination and integration. Students could work on the development of cross-agency outcome measures for children and families that would form the basis of service planning, coordination, and outcome evaluation. Also, students could provide information for local legislators on the difficult choices about which mixture of services and benefits to fund and summarize research-based knowledge as one input in the decision process.

ASSESSING LEARNING IN COMMUNITIES OF PRACTICE

The community of practice surrounding field study in social policy programs is only complete when knowledge is shared among students, faculty, and field participants, and learning is assessed in relation to formal and tacit knowledge sources. Knowledge sharing and assessment are mutually reinforcing and require a direct interplay between formalized and tacit knowledge, representing the academic and practitioner communities respectively. Three strategies for sharing and assessing field-study learning—project specific concept maps, a generic knowledge classification structure, and a research and curriculum development project on tacit knowledge relevant to applied developmental science—will be described that illustrate different ways of making more explicit the interplay between academic and field-based sources of knowledge.

Concept Maps

As described above, concept maps are one practical means of accomplishing both the knowledge sharing and assessment tasks. As described by Novak and Gowin (1984), concept maps can be evaluated in terms of their structure and content. For example, Figure 4.3 shows a concept map developed by a team of undergraduates in a social policy research methods course based on literature review, observation through field placement in a drug treatment agency, and interviews with human

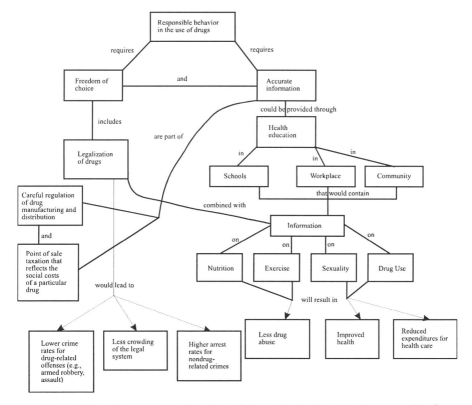

Figure 4.3 A Concept Map Developed through Field Study of Drug Policy.[2]

service and law enforcement professionals. The causal arguments about the effects of legalizing drugs in combination with education, regulation and taxation policies reflected one perspective drawn from research literature and professional opinion. Other maps noted gaps in knowledge (e.g., rates of abuse or addiction among the general population under legalization in relation to specific substances) as well as the harmful effects of current policies of law enforcement and adjudication on children and families.

Evaluation of a concept map's structure focuses on the relationships among concepts and whether they are organized appropriately in terms of categories and their components (e.g., nutrition and sexuality are part of education programs), lateral relationships among concepts (e.g., the significance of regulation done in parallel with education), and the definition of specific concepts (e.g., point-of-sale taxation designation). Each concept and relationship can form the basis of exam questions, should require further elaboration in terms of tacit and/or research knowledge, and can be assessed through written, oral, visual or other formats. In this way, concept maps provide an explicit basis for students to demonstrate their understanding of knowledge structures and sources.

Given that field study can involve demonstration of skilled performance—for example, interning in a drug treatment program, designing an evaluation of a health education program—some part of knowledge sharing and assessment should involve analysis of caregiving, research methods and other situation specific expertise, with significant input from field mentors. The role of off-campus professionals who serve as internship supervisors or project clients is important in assessing the degree to which student skills that have been presented in the classroom, such as program evaluation methods, are effective in the field community of practice. For example, health education outcome measures that represent sound psychometric properties may be too costly or may not reflect important program, client or community goals. Similarly, concepts maps can form the basis of learning contracts in which students and faculty identify the content and skill development to be obtained from field study.

Concept maps are also useful for sharing knowledge among faculty, students and field participants. One application of concept maps in the veterinary medical sciences at Cornell University described how they were publicly posted by faculty so that the knowledge structures and learning objectives could be shared with students and colleagues alike (Edmondson & Smith, 1996). Used in this fashion, concept maps enliven knowledge sharing which is integral to the very notion of communities of practice.

Another way of using concept maps for assessing learning is to link them to pedagogical frameworks such as Kolb's (1984) four phase model of experience, reflection, abstraction, and experimentation. Faculty and field mentors might evaluate each learning phase in ways suited to learner strengths as follows: 1) review literature and conduct field-based observations and interviews in drug treatment and enforcement settings (experience); 2) distill formal and tacit knowledge into concepts (reflection); 3) formalize knowledge into a concept map with defined interrelationships among concepts (abstraction); and 4) develop practitioner and research-based methods for testing aspects of the concept map (experimentation).

Forms of Knowledge

A second approach to teaching and assessment of learning in field study is derived from Shulman's (1986) work on different forms of knowledge used by teachers in their professional practice. His framework is a general one that can be applied to many professions and consists of three categories—propositional, case, and strategic knowledge.

Within propositional forms of knowledge, Shulman identifies three subcategories as shown below:

4. Propositional knowledge—cause and effect or moral principle statements intended to influence specific situations faced by professional.
   a. Knowledge derived from theory and research.
      Example—In the workplace, subordinates seldom volunteer negative feedback to their superiors.
   b. Knowledge derived from experience in the form of practical maxims.
      Example—The additional time taken to reach consensus on a decision is usually worth the cost compared to trying to overcome the resistance to implementing the decision.
   c. Knowledge derived from ethics or moral principles.
      Example—Organizations should have a social responsibility for the well-being of their employees and the larger society within which they exist.

Shulman's second general category is referred to as case knowledge. The value of case knowledge in terms of student learning is that it makes propositional knowledge more memorable, since the latter typically consists of very long lists, and provides context that helps the practitioner consider which situations are most appropriate for the application of propositions. Case methods of teaching are designed to employ the vivid detail of field situations but to do so in the service of exemplifying more general theoretical or normative points. These general points must be drawn from reflection and interpretation since the case itself is only descriptive of a particular situation. Because of its generalizing purpose, the power of case knowledge resides in the number and diversity of analogous situations to which it can be applied.

Case knowledge also has three subcategories in Shulman's framework parallel to propositional knowledge (but in case study, not propositional, form) as follows:

5. Case knowledge
   a. Prototype knowledge which exemplifies theoretical ideas or underlying mechanisms.
      Example—A case that illustrated how negative behavior is often inadvertently reinforced.
   b. Precedent knowledge representing principles of professional practice.
      Example—A case that described how to avoid calling attention to disruptive behavior in the classroom.
   c. Parable knowledge which conveys norms and values.
      Example—A case that reinforced the value of taking responsibility for one's behavior.

A given case can represent one or more of these subcategories. Typically cases are formulated as precedent knowledge in that they are based on actual examples of professional or organizational behavior. Prototype cases also are used in most disciplines, however, not because they represent frequent or even actual situations, but because they illustrate theoretical principles. Examples would include psychoanalytic cases in psychotherapy that portray general principles of client-therapist relations, or descriptions of idealized markets to illustrate economic principles of perfect competition.

The following abbreviated case adapted from Shulman (1986) illustrates each type of case knowledge.

48

Social Change, Public Policy, and Community Collaborations: Training
Human Development Professionals for the Twenty-First Century

> Several students repeatedly come to school without a pencil and thus are unable to do class work. The teacher could supply pencils or "punish" the students by having them sit through class and do the work later (but they would just fall further behind). Both of these approaches risk reinforcing negative behavior, calling attention to disruptive behavior, and absolving the students of responsibility. The teacher's solution was to keep a box of very short pencils that have to be used to do all the day's work by students who do not come prepared. (p. 12)

Both propositional and case knowledge are applied to or learned in relation to a specific situation. It is difficult to remember a large number of propositions unless they are organized in some conceptual framework or hierarchy that allows for groupings of content from the more specific to the more general. Case knowledge begins to address that need and is intended to support generalizations, but it has to be explicitly linked to underlying concepts or principles that can be applied to new situations.

These limitations lead to Shulman's (1986) third category which he calls "strategic knowledge," although as he notes, it may be more appropriate to think of this category as a process than a form of knowledge. The following quotation should make clear why strategic knowledge requires an appreciation of the learning process itself:

> Strategic knowledge must be generated to extend understanding beyond principle to the wisdom of practice. We generally attribute wisdom to those who can transcend the limitations of particular principles or specific experiences when confronted by situations in which each of the alternative choices appears equally 'principled.' . . . The professional holds knowledge, not only of how—the capacity for skilled performance—but of what and why. . . . [Strategic] knowledge guarantees only grounded unpredictability, the exercise of reasoned judgment, rather than the display of correct behavior. (p. 13)

These descriptions of strategic knowledge are very similar to what Schön (1983) refers to as reflection-in-action and professional artistry. Knowledge exists in many forms that sometimes can be arrayed along continua such as predictable to unpredictable, explicit to implicit, public to private, unidimensional to multidimensional, rule-based expertise to improvisational artistry, and technical skill to wisdom.

It is tempting to label one kind of knowledge as more sophisticated or valuable than another, yet different types of knowledge can be equally useful depending on the demands of the situation. Learning must consist of the content of a discipline or field (e.g., as described in the previous section for the social policy curriculum), its propositions, theories, and methods of knowledge creation and professional practice. Strategic knowledge, however, because it is dealing with less determinate situations and the application of reasoned judgment more than skilled performance, reflects a process of learning more than factual content. Strategic knowledge virtually requires experiential and field-based forms of pedagogy that are created under a vision of communities of practice.

Tacit Knowledge Research and Curriculum Development

A third approach to assessing student learning in the community of practice framework for field study is illustrated through a research and curriculum development project on which the author is participating. Its purposes are to: 1) identify relationships between research-based and practitioner-based knowledge in the development of professional expertise; and 2) develop concept mapping methods for assessing student knowledge that link classroom and experiential learning (e.g., through clinical internships and field study).

The research design assesses the effects of different instructional conditions that vary the linkages between didactic (research-based) and experiential (practitioner-based) learning within veterinary medicine and management, two fields with contrasting research bases (natural vs. social sciences) and fundamental practice demands (clinical vs. social). Within each profession several broad content areas are identified to serve as the focus of knowledge transformation (e.g., inter-agency collaboration for management; radiographic interpretation for medicine). Initial interviews are conducted with cooperating faculty and professional experts in order to: 1) identify key concepts in each content area; 2) develop maps that depict the conceptual structures for the content area; and 3) develop descriptions of routine and complex problems that require knowledge of those concept structures. The concept maps are used as baselines to assess students' concept map attributes in ways that validly represent research-based and practitioner-based knowledge for solving or addressing the routine and complex problems in each focal area.

This project attempts to overcome a feature of experiential learning that can inhibit the adoption of field study by a broader array of faculty: the lack of specificity on content area knowledge that forms the basis for teaching and for assessing learning. It seeks to overcome this limitation by developing course-specific content and methods for assessing learning. In these ways, it is hoped that the intellectual value of experiential learning will be clarified and field study will become integrated with a wider array of courses in the curriculum.

Each of these three approaches to assessing learning in communities of practice—concept maps, forms of knowledge, and tacit knowledge research—requires substantial investment in faculty and curriculum development if the knowledge to be gained from integrating field and classroom learning is to be adequately defined. Approaches as comprehensive as these must be pursued, however, in order to specify knowledge and learning goals and thereby give field study an intellectual status comparable to that of traditional classroom pedagogy.

CONCLUSION

Ultimately, the knowledge assessment questions raised with respect to field study in applied developmental science transcend particular subject matter. They have to do with developing students' capacity for applied theorizing in three ways: 1) the ability to conceptualize disparate bits of information from subject matter and experience into clusters, concepts, and relationships, and to reframe these conceptualizations by changing perspectives and assumptions; 2) the ability to formulate and test hypotheses, especially by finding field study opportunities to experience and examine subject matter concepts; and 3) the ability to use value conflict, ambiguity of problem definition, and uncertainty about the efficacy of interventions as a source of exploration and knowledge development (McClintock, 1990a). Collaboration between the campus and the community is essential for engaging students in this kind of meaningful learning and research on the complex and often dramatic challenges of concern to applied developmental science such as access to affordable and quality health care, effective education for all children, and the multifaceted topics of employment, child care and family functioning flowing from welfare reform.

Creating communities of field-based practice in policy studies as a means of motivating and enriching student learning is not an easy or inexpensive effort. It requires investment in faculty development and professional mentors to integrate field-based activity into more traditional lecture and discussion classroom settings. And it requires a commitment to communities of learning which, as Palmer (1987) puts it, represent "a capacity for relatedness within individuals—relatedness not only to people but to events in history, to nature, to the world of ideas, and yes, to things of the spirit" (p. 24). If this approach to experiential learning achieves positive results in terms of subject matter learning and developing student capacities for applied theorizing, it is well worth the effort and adds distinctive value to policy studies in applied developmental science.

NOTES

I wish to gratefully acknowledge the useful comments from Ann Mullis on an earlier version of this chapter presented at the Third National Conference on Applied Developmental Science, Florida State University, College of Human Sciences, Tallahassee, FL, March 1997.
1. Tacit knowledge can reside in the classroom or in the field. Its defining characteristic is that it is knowledge for which there is less explication and support in learning (Williams & Sternberg, 1997). For example, when teaching students how to conduct policy and program evaluation research, faculty will emphasize empirical and analytic technique over what might be termed the "artistry" or conceptual dimension of conducting research for a sponsoring client. In a practicum, students might be expected to absorb lessons about the messiness of actually doing evaluation research, but there are few guides for formalizing the more discretionary aspects of it (McGrath, Martin & Kulka, 1982).
2. Responsible behavior in the use of drugs required freedom of choice and accurate information. Free choice includes the legalization of drugs, while accurate information could be provided through health education in the schools, the workplace and the community. Careful regulation of drug manufacturing and distribution and point-of-sale taxation that reflects the social costs of a particular drug are also part of accurate information. Legalization of drugs under these conditions would lead to lower crime rates for drug-related offenses (e.g., armed robbery), less crowding of the legal system, and higher arrest rates for non-drug-related crimes. Legalization, combined with education programs that contain information on nutrition, exercise, sexuality and drug use, would also result in less drug abuse, improved health, and reduced expenditures for health care.

REFERENCES

Anderson, C. W. (1993). *Prescribing the life of the mind.* Madison, WI: University of Wisconsin Press.
Averch, H. & Dluhy, M. (1992). Teaching public administration, public management, and policy analysis: Convergence or divergence in the masters core. *Journal of Policy Analysis and Management, 11,* 541-551.
Bensimon, E. M. & Soto, M. (1997). Can we rebuild civic life without a multiracial university? *Change, 29,* 42-44.
Boyer, E. L. (1990). *Scholarship reconsidered: Priorities of the professoriate.* Princeton, NJ: The Carnegie Foundation for the Advancement of Teaching.
Boyer, E. L. (1994, March 9). The new American college. *Chronicle of Higher Education,* A-48.
Bronfenbrenner, U. (1979). *The ecology of human development: Experiments by nature and design.* Cambridge, MA: Harvard University Press.
Bronfenbrenner, U., McClelland, P., Wethington, E., Moen, P. & Ceci, S. J. (1996). *The state of Americans: This generation and the next.* New York: Free Press.
Brown, J. S., Collins, A. & Duguid, S. (1989). Situated cognition and the culture of learning. *Educational Researcher, 18,* 32-42.
College of Human Ecology. (1994). *Foundations of excellence.* Ithaca, NY: Cornell University.
Dewey, J. (1986). Logic: The theory of inquiry. In J. A. Boydston (Ed.), *John Dewey: The later works, 1925-1953, Vol. 12.* Carbondale: Southern Illinois University Press. (Original work published 1938).

Edmondson, K. M. & Smith, D. F. (1996). Concept mapping to facilitate veterinary students' understanding of fluid and electrolyte disorders. Paper presented at the annual meeting of the American Educational Research Association, New York, NY.

Etzioni, A. (Ed.). (1995). *New communitarian thinking: Persons, virtues, institutions and communities.* Charlottesville: University of Virginia Press.

Gamson, Z. F. (1997). Higher education and rebuilding civic life. *Change, 29,* 10-13.

Gardner, H. (1993). *Multiple intelligences: The theory in practice.* New York: Basic Books.

Hamilton, S. (1990). *Apprenticeship for adulthood: Preparing youth for the future.* New York: Free Press.

Hutchings, P. & Wutzdorff, A. (Eds.). (1988). *Knowing and doing: Learning through experience. New directions for teaching and learning, Vol. 35.* San Francisco: Jossey-Bass.

Jacoby, B. & Associates. (Eds.). (1996). *Service-learning in higher education: Concepts and practices.* San Francisco: Jossey-Bass

Kennedy, M. M. (1997). The connection between research and practice. *Educational Researcher, 26,* 4-12.

Knowles, M. (1984). *Andragogy in action.* San Francisco: Jossey-Bass.

Kolb, D. A. (1984). *Experiential learning.* Englewood Cliffs, NJ: Prentice-Hall.

Lave, J. & Wenger, E. (1991). *Situated learning: Legitimate peripheral participation.* Cambridge, England: Cambridge University Press.

Lerner, R. M. & Fisher, C. B. (1994). From applied developmental psychology to applied developmental science: Community coalitions and collaborative careers. In C. B. Fisher & R. M. Lerner (Eds.) *Applied developmental psychology* (pp. 505-522). New York: McGraw-Hill.

McClintock, C. (1999). Policy seminars for state and community leaders. In T. Chibucos and R. Lerner (Eds.) *Serving children and families through community-university partnerships: Success stories* (pp. 269-274). Norwell, MA: Kluwer.

McClintock, C. (1996). (Ed.). *Academic plan for the creation of the department of policy analysis and management in the College of Human Ecology, Cornell University.* Ithaca, NY: New York State College of Human Ecology, Cornell University

McClintock, C. (1994). (Ed.). *Foundations of excellence—College of Human Ecology strategic planning report.* Ithaca, NY: New York State College of Human Ecology, Cornell University.

McClintock, C. (1990a). A common thread: Teaching students to think theoretically. *Human Ecology Forum, 18,* 12-15.

McClintock, C. (1990b). Evaluators as applied theorists. *Evaluation Practice, 11,* 1-14.

McClintock, C. & Beck, S. (1998). Multicultural education in urban affairs: Field-based learning about diversity. *Journal of Family and Consumer Sciences, 90*(1), 49-53.

McClintock, C. & Colosi, L. (1998). Evaluating welfare reform: A framework for including the urgent and the important. *Evaluation Review, 22,* 668-694.

McGrath, J. E., Martin, J. & Kulka, R. A. (1982). *Judgment calls in research.* Beverly Hills, CA: Sage.

Moore, D. T. (1990). Experiential education as critical discourse. In J. C. Kendall and Associates (Eds.) *Combining Service and Learning: A Resource Book for Community and Public Service, Vol. 1.* Raleigh, NC: National Society for Experiential Education.

Novak, J. D. & Gowin, D. B. (1984). *Learning how to learn.* Cambridge, England: Cambridge University Press.

Palmer, P. J. (1987). Community, conflict, and ways of knowing: Ways to deepen our educational agenda. *Change, 19,* 20-25.

Rifkin, J. (1995). *The end of work: The decline of the global labor force and the dawn of the post-market era.* New York: Tarcher/Putnam.

Schön, D. A. (1983). *The reflective practitioner: How professionals think in action.* New York: Basic Books.

Schön, D. A. (1987). *Educating the reflective practitioner.* San Francisco: Jossey-Bass.

Shulman, L. S. (1986, February). Those who understand: Knowledge growth in teaching. *Educational Researcher,* 4-14.

Sirianni, C. & Friedland, L. (1997). Civic innovation and American democracy. *Change, 29,* 14-23.

Stanton, T. K. & Giles, D. E. (1989). Curriculum development for long-distance internships: Some principles, models and issues. In S. W. Weil & I. McGill (Eds.), *Making sense of experiential learning.* Philadelphia: Society for Research into Higher Education and Open University Press.

Sternberg, R. J. (1985). *Beyond IQ.* New York: Cambridge University Press.

Williams, W. M. & Sternberg, R. J. (1997). *Success acts for managers.* Orlando, FL: Harcourt Brace.

Antidotes for Arrogance: Training Applied Developmental Scientists in Public Policy Contexts

Brian L. Wilcox, *University of Nebraska-Lincoln*

I am delighted to have this opportunity to outline the issues surrounding field training for human developmental professionals in public policy settings. Both in my current position at the University of Nebraska's Center on Children, Families, and the Law and in my former position as Director of Public Policy at the American Psychological Association, I have directed public policy internship programs for pre- and post-doctoral psychologists with interests in child and family policy. I believe that direct policy experience can benefit our students in a wide variety of ways, but I have always believed that the prime benefit of such direct encounters with the policy world is that they can serve as a powerful antidote to professional arrogance. In this chapter, I will explain first what I mean by this, and then will present one picture of what field training in public policy might look like.

SOURCES OF PROFESSIONAL ARROGANCE

Deep within many of our disciplines is a disdain for politics and all things political. Politics are seen as a corrupting influence by many in the academic world. Professionals who work in policy contexts are sometimes seen as being in a league with the devil. This is especially true the closer one gets to the political side of the policy world. About 12 years ago I decided to take a leave from my faculty position to spend a year as a Congressional Science Fellow working in the office of a member of Congress. The fellowship was sponsored by the Society for Research in Child Development, and obtaining the fellowship required going through a fairly grueling competition. I thought that receiving this fellowship was quite an honor until I mentioned it to my psychology department colleagues at the University of Virginia. Their responses were . . . well, interesting. They mainly ran from bemused to appalled. "That's certainly a different thing to do with your time," replied one colleague to my news. "Are you out of your [expletive deleted] mind?" commented one of my friends in the experimental psychology area. Only a couple had any appreciation of the potential value of the fellowship experience. Many of our colleagues have some appreciation that policy and politics have some bearing on our professional lives, and a smaller subset seem to agree that there is value (and even virtue) in our interacting with the policy world, but few regard policy involvement in any form as central to our professional identity.

To many, the world of policy and politics are at least marginally familiar. We read about policy issues in our papers and watch coverage of political and policy matters on television. Some have gone so far as to watch C-SPAN's coverage of some policy proceedings. This familiarity with the "surface structure" of policy and politics gives some an illusory sense that they understand the "deep structure." In other words, this sense of familiarity gives some of our colleagues a feeling that they really understand the policy process. This form of arrogance is, of course, common. Many policy makers, for example, believe that they understand child development because they were children once, after all, and isn't it all just 'common sense' anyway? The point here is that most academic developmentalists, even those with very applied interests, have a very limited understanding of the complexities of the public policy process and, more importantly, don't fully appreciate the limits of their understanding.

For this book, I have been asked to address issues relating to field training of applied developmental scientists in the area of public policy. I am very pleased that the editors have seen fit to include this issue, as it has been my experience that field training is often an afterthought in graduate programs where public policy is a secondary focus.

Let me begin by stating that I believe that field training in public policy is essential to graduate training in applied developmental science, and especially so in programs that claim to offer students an emphasis on the relationship between developmental science and public policy. Field training grounds the academic training we provide our students and is perhaps the most powerful antidote to professional arrogance of the type I have described.

One more prefatory comment is needed before we turn to public policy field training issues. One of the most common forms of professional arrogance I have seen in applied human development programs is faculty's propensity to send students into policy field placements with no didactic policy training. One program I visited was pleased that they had placed a number of graduate students in the offices of several state legislators. When I spoke with the students, however, they felt that they had been poorly prepared for the experience and consequently came away with much less from a promising experience than should have been the case. As one student noted, "I spent the first five weeks completely lost because I didn't understand a thing about what they were doing in the committee I worked with." Knowing little of the policy process or the language of policy making, the students were left to their own devices to grasp the complexities of policy making in an environment where no one was likely to have the time to sit down with them and explain the facts of legislative life.

Think of this situation another way. Would an accounting program send its students into businesses before learning the basic principles of accounting? Would we allow students to be placed in a family therapy or spouse abuse clinic if they hadn't received proper training? I think not, but that is precisely what I have found we often do with students wanting to be placed in a policy setting. I believe quite strongly that it is inappropriate and quite possibly unethical for us to send students into settings without providing them adequate preparation.

PUBLIC POLICY FIELD EXPERIENCES

I will devote most of this chapter to describing the varieties of field training which might be instituted by graduate programs in applied developmental science, but I would like to briefly touch on the rationale for training human development professionals in public policy contexts. I will state this rationale as simply as possible using Urie Bronfenbrenner's (1974) arguments: engaging students in the public policy arena brings both vitality and validity to applied developmental science. Giving students the opportunity to apply their coursework in a setting where decisions make a difference in the lives of children and families reinforces what they've learned, brings it to life in a way that can't be done using didactic teaching methods, and provides an excellent testing ground for our theories. Working in such settings can also give our students a glimpse of the limitations of our knowledge. There are many important questions bearing directly on the lives of children and families that we have not yet begun to address. Knowing the limitations of our knowledge as we attempt to help policy makers solve real problems is perhaps the most powerful antidote to professional arrogance.

There are a wide variety of types of settings within which graduate students can be usefully placed to gain policy experiences related to human development issues. By policy experiences, I am referring to placement in settings in which policy is made, informed, or influenced. I define policy as a process or as a set of decisions rather than as a singular decision such as the passage of legislation. The process, and the set of decisions, run from defining a problem or issue as one warranting the attention of policy makers to evaluating the consequences of policy implementation and feeding those findings back into the policy process. There are opportunities for field training across all points in the policy process.

Let's consider the policy process as portrayed in Figure 5.1. The first stage in this process is labeled "Problems to Government" and refers to the process of problem perception and definition. Perhaps the key way that developmentalists can influence this part of the policy process is by conducting targeted policy-oriented research intended to highlight the nature of a problem, such as child maltreatment, or more generally the problems affecting children. With respect to field training possibilities, there are numerous activities that can provide students with this type of experience. In Nebraska we have placed students with two different policy advocacy organizations that conduct primary and secondary research intended to mobilize action in the state legislature. One organization, Voices for Children-Nebraska, conducts the state's annual "Kids Count" survey. One of our students assisted the organization with this project. Another student worked with a local public interest law group to analyze the likely effects of welfare reform on the state's poor children. This student summarized the research on the consequences of poverty on child development and helped develop the model predicting the number of Nebraska children likely to be affected by various aspects of the welfare reform legislation. Other students have worked on research examining the predictors of child abuse reporting and case substantiation, with the goal of informing social services policy.

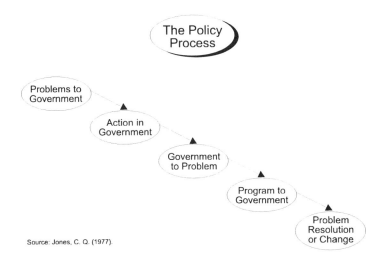

Source: Jones, C. Q. (1977).

Figure 5.1 The Policy Process.

There are a number of skills students normally acquire in this type of setting. First, students begin to learn more about the policy process without being thoroughly enmeshed in it. Second, students learn how to frame questions in ways that are appropriately directed to policy questions. Third, students often acquire new research skills that are more characteristically used in policy research than traditional developmental research. Finally, students learn how to write up the results of their work for policy consumers and the media.

The second stage of the policy process is labeled "Action in Government" and refers to policy formulation and the legislative process, including both authorization and appropriation. There are a number of avenues for involvement in the legislative process. Field training opportunities exist in legislative committee offices, the individual offices of legislators, in legislative support offices (which would include policy research units like the General Accounting Office or the Congressional Research Service), and with external organizations which work to influence the legislative process.

Students placed in legislative settings must be well-versed in the policy process, generally, and more specifically in the legislative process. Our students who have worked in state and federal legislative offices have mainly functioned in roles where they attempt to "translate" social science research for the policy makers with whom they work. There is little opportunity for conducting research in these environments, but students have found numerous instances in which they are able to bring their developmental training directly to bear on a policy issue.

When placing students in a legislative setting, it is important to bear in mind that their experiences will be largely dictated by events not under their control. The legislative process can be unpredictable, and students who enter settings thinking they will be working on one issue might find themselves working on nearly everything but that issue. For example, one student I know of spent a semester working almost exclusively on veterans affairs issues. He learned a great deal about the legislative process and the politics surrounding this policy area. While he did not apply his developmental training directly, he found the experience to be, on the whole, a worthwhile one.

The best legislative placements, however, allow students to work on issues relevant to their training. Placing students in the offices of committees with jurisdiction of child welfare issues, for example, is a good way of improving the odds that this will occur. Committee staff tend to have a far more focused portfolio of issues to cover than is the case for staff working in the offices of individual members of the legislature.

The third stage of the policy process is labeled "Government to Problem" and refers to the process of the development of regulations and program implementation. This part of the process typically takes place within government agencies and not the legislative bodies. Once a piece of legislation is passed, government agencies assume the task of developing the regulations governing the program created by the legislation and then implementing the program.

Students can learn a fundamental policy lesson by working in an agency that has the task of developing regulations and implementing programs, especially if the student has had an opportunity to follow the legislation over time. In this type of setting students learn that those who develop regulations and implement programs either are given or often assume considerable discretion in the way they interpret the statute directing their work. That is, both the regulations guiding the program and the actual implementation of the program may vary significantly from the original intent of the legislature. This "slip between the cup and the lip" is a time-honored practice in public policy and has been studied extensively by political scientists (e.g., see Pressman & Wildavsky, 1973). Understanding the flow of events from legislative action to regulations to implementation is critical in gaining a complete understanding of the policy process. Seeing this disjuncture take place is always more informative than reading about it.

Students placed in administrative agencies can sometimes find themselves caught up in the mundane day-to-day activities of the agency, with little opportunity to connect what they are doing and seeing to the larger policy process. It is essential that students in any placement, but especially those in administrative settings, have routine supervision.

The fourth stage of the policy process, and the last we will be concerned with, is referred to as "Program to Government." This part of the process encompasses the efforts of the agencies and the legislature to determine whether the actions they have taken to address the problem formulated in the first stage of the policy process are effective or make sense. Various policy analysis tools, including program evaluation and benefit/cost analysis among others, may be utilized by both agency personnel, researchers under contract with the government, and/or privately funded researchers to determine the direction and/or fate of a given program. Students can be placed with any organization undertaking this policy analysis/evaluation role. In some cases, universities have research centers which carry out such work. My center, the Center on Children, Families, and the Law at the University of Nebraska, has evaluation projects funded either by the federal or state governments or by private foundations which are assessing the effectiveness of programs created by legislative action. We involve a number of students in these projects.

This type of placement is often the most comfortable for faculty supervisors because they can easily relate to the activities taking place. It is important to keep in mind, however, that evaluation research taking place within a policy context must be managed very carefully. There are frequently a number of powerful stakeholders who are keenly interested in the results. Care must be taken not only in the way the research is conducted but also in the way the results are communicated, Much will be made of who is informed, when they are informed, how they are informed, and who is not informed. Missteps can be very costly, and this kind of "research in a fishbowl" requires special administrative and political skills than can be very useful to the student interested in public policy.

In summary, there is a vast array of potential policy settings within which students can acquire useful skills and knowledge. It is my belief that students wishing to specialize in the relationship between applied developmental science and public policy should try to gain experience in settings across the policy process in order to gain a more complete sense of that process in operation. Students with a less central interest in public policy can profit from a single placement provided that they receive supervision which helps them integrate their experiences and understand how they fit into the broader policy process.

SUPERVISION

Supervision, in my thinking, is the key to successful field placements, yet it is often overlooked and underdeveloped. In my discussions with applied developmental science students who have had policy placements, their most common complaint was with the lack of supervision they received. Several reported receiving no supervision at all, suggesting that the faculty treated the placement more like a job than a learning experience,

Being a developmentalist in a policy setting can be a bit like being a fish out of water. Many of the people you are working with do not quite know what to make of you. They may be unsure of what your skills are or what you might contribute. This is especially true in settings associated with policy formulation and implementation. Students in these situations need both guidance and reassurance. Students need assistance in determining how their experiences clarify the policy process and the relationship of social science knowledge to that process. Students will occasionally need advice on how to handle delicate political issues that they have never before confronted.

The central goal of supervision should be the integration of the experience with coursework and with the goals of the graduate program. I have found that supervision works best when there are regular meetings involving not only the student and the faculty supervisor but also a supervisor in the field placement. This allows for regular communication between program faculty and field placement staff to assure that the needs of both parties are being well served. Problems can be headed off early and opportunities being missed can be identified.

CONCLUSION

Field placements in public policy settings should be treated like any other element in our graduate curriculum. We should begin by asking why we are asking students to complete them. What do these placements contribute to the students' education? Where do they fit within the curriculum? What prerequisites are necessary or appropriate to maximize their benefit to the students? Who should supervise the students and what qualifications should the supervisors have? We should have the answers to questions such as these before we implement public policy field training. Poorly implemented field experiences benefit no one and carry a risk of alienating both students and policy makers. Soundly designed and implemented field experience programs, on the other hand, can give students an array of valuable skills and help build stronger bridges between our programs and policy makers. Given that the stakes can be quite high, it is essential that we take the high road and do it right.

REFERENCES

Bronfenbrenner, U. (1974). Developmental research and public policy. In J. M. Romanyshyn (Ed.), *Social science and social welfare*. New York: Council of Social Work Education.
Jones, C. O. (1977). *An introduction to the study of public policy* (2nd ed.). Belmont, CA: Wadsworth.
Pressman, J. L. & Wildavsky, A. B. (1973). *Implementation: How great expectations in Washington are dashed in Oakland; or, why it's amazing that Federal programs work at all*. Berkeley, CA: University of California Press.

As We Sow . . . A Pragmatic Analysis of How to Build Successful Partnerships between the University and the Larger Community

Bea Smith, *University of Missouri-Columbia*

PROLOGUE

Last August, to my surprise and delight, the Columbia Garden Club pounded a rather impressive sign in my front yard proclaiming it to be our community's Yard of the Month, and I was invited to share my success secrets at a Garden Club luncheon. Here, I have been invited to discuss the changing of university culture to foster collaboration with the larger community. In many respects, the processes are remarkably similar.

When I was in eighth grade, the Iowa legislature decided that all Iowa kids should know about enlightened farming practices. The simple lessons, field trips to terraced fields, and awkward explanations by sunburned men in seed corn company caps left a lasting impression useful for both urban gardening and academic administration. I learned that one cannot simply broadcast seeds and expect a bountiful harvest to rightfully come one's way. One has to start with fertile soil or to enhance the soil, which must then be carefully cultivated according to good conservation practices so there is not undue leaching or runoff, with an obligation to leave a fertile legacy for future generations. Crops are carefully planned and rotated. Poor quality seed is a bad choice even if it's a lot cheaper. Fertilizer is applied judiciously—the right kind, the right quantity, the right timing. One can *assist*, but not *control* weather and other fates, so there's always an element of capriciousness. Work-sharing with neighbors lightens tasks. Planning for the next season is on-going. The results of the previous season do not foreordain the present to either failure or bounty. And, at the church on the corner, we were taught to give thanks for the harvest, knowing well that sweat equity complemented divine benevolence.

We learned a work and responsibility ethic. Most of us also heard the moralistic tale of the workmen who are interviewed about their activities on a project far removed from rural Iowa. One says matter-of-factly that he's mixing cement. Another, that he's building a wall. And still another, while gazing rapturously toward far horizons, exalts, "I'm building a cathedral!" The message, of course, is that the most mundane tasks can be ennobled if one has a vision. Pragmatically, however, if the cathedral is to soar skyward and endure, the subsoil must be firm, the cement of good quality and the walls in plumb. Vision alone is not enough.

The special role that has been charted for this chapter is a pragmatic analysis of how to develop successful partnerships—changing, as necessary, the university culture to foster collaboration. Academics often seem to apologize for a pragmatic orientation, as though the term is antithetical to their roles and well-being. The result is too often imprisonment in the ivory tower of public perception. But the

60

*Social Change, Public Policy, and Community Collaborations: Training
Human Development Professionals for the Twenty-First Century*

pragmatic approach, defined as "relating to the affairs of a community or state . . .
practical . . . dealing with events in such a manner as to show their interconnection,"
is the engine of success in getting things done for the university within the larger
community. The ideas that follow will seek to legitimize political pragmatism for
the new American scholar in a human development discipline. They are predicated
on needs charted by distinguished academicians, grounded in action strategies and
advice from legislators and agency heads who must grapple with conflicting
pressures, and encouraged by legislative liaisons and public relations officers who
are charged with selling and humanizing the university culture to various publics.

THE VISION: EDUCATIONAL INSTITUTIONS THAT ARE RELEVANT
TO SOCIETAL NEEDS

The specific purpose of the conference that served as the basis for this book was to
change the character of graduate and undergraduate education in the human
development-related disciplines by developing curricula and identifying a cadre of
educators who will prepare the next generation of scholars for public policy
engagement. None too soon! Derek Bok, from the bully pulpit of the Harvard
University presidency, wrote, "Observing our difficulties competing abroad, our
millions of people in poverty, our drug-ridden communities, our disintegrating
families, our ineffective schools, those who help to shape our universities have
reason to ask whether they too have any time to lose" (Bok, 1990, cover).
Discussing whether or not universities are doing *enough* to build civic
responsibility, ethical awareness, and economic competitiveness, Bok lamented that
"we lead most industrial democracies in ignorance and in many of the pathologies
of modern civilization while lagging behind in the rate of economic progress" (p. 6).
And yet, the premise that universities should realign their priorities to address social
problems is not universally accepted:

> Such critics look approvingly on earlier conceptions of the
> academy . . . a place detached from society, uncontaminated by its
> worldly values, and undistracted by pursuits other than the search
> for greater knowledge and understanding . . . It would be a pity,
> however, if an insistence on pure learning and research were to
> drive out all concern for practical issues. Not only does society
> need the university's help to solve many of its problems, such
> problems can also help scholars to discern more basic questions
> and to acquire practical experience that casts new light on familiar
> issues. Besides, the division between pure and instrumental
> inquiry is much too sharp. It is possible to explore a subject out of
> a keen desire to understand it better *and* a belief that such
> understanding may be of use to humankind . . . One would
> suppose, therefore, that the true mission of universities would be
> to nurture a healthy balance between applied intellectual pursuits
> and the search for truth and meaning for their own sake. (Bok,
> 1990, pp. 7-10)

The pragmatic importance of connecting the inquiry and knowledge of the
university to social problems was bannered in a headline in *The Columbia (MO)
Daily Tribune* that trumpeted, "Senator Throws Prison Challenge at UM." The
article linked the flat higher education budget recommendation of a pro-education
governor to other funding priorities. "Senators told [interim University president]
George the cost of new prisons is cutting into money for colleges" (Keller, 1997, p.

1). The chairman of the House appropriations committee, pointing out that $170 million had been earmarked for new prisons, with additional millions set aside to pay for guards, said, "We'd have a lot more money if you could tell us how to keep from building more prisons in this state. We need help from academia. Finding a solution could be one of the best things you could do for higher education in this state in terms of making additional money available" (p. 1). Could there be a clearer clarion call to academics on the cause-and-effect relationship between socially relevant work and future support?

John Lombardi, president of the University of Florida, speaking to land-grant lay leaders, expressed the quandary and the challenge:

> What a time we live in! Nothing remains stable, nothing stays the same, and even those of us who work in universities find ourselves under intense pressure to change, reform and restructure. Our budgets come under attack from legislators pressed to find funds for crime prevention, health care, and public schools; our hold on the popular imagination weakens as some of our colleagues cut corners and betray our trust; our claim to serve the needs of our students appears hollow as we find it necessary to filter out students we don't have the room to educate. On every side we find critics eager to attack the university, eager to demonstrate our failings in undergraduate education, enthusiastic in pointing out our inability to reward teaching in our large universities, and caustic in their dismissal of the real challenges universities face. (Lombardi, 1992, p. 1)

Universities contain the wherewithal to make a difference in areas of humanistic and economic needs. But are they effectively mustering their resources to address the needs and assuage those critics? As Derek Bok prepared to leave the Harvard presidency, he lamented to a reporter, "You are struck by what an inverse correlation there is between what society needs from these institutions and what we are taking most seriously. If you take some of the basic problems facing our society . . . and then make a list of all the things that a university could contribute . . . and ask yourself how do all these things rank in the list of priorities of the modern university, one is struck by how low they rank. [For example,] when poverty, homelessness, drug abuse and chronic unemployment are major problems, schools of social work are neglected and, like faculties of education, they are poor stepchildren on most university campuses" (Goldman, 1990, p. A5).

Many in the human development professions rue the reality of being those poor stepchildren and ask how they can have impact on those priorities. As Bok suggests, the challenge is to make a case for "a healthy balance between applied intellectual pursuits and the search for truth and meaning for their own sake" (p. 10). Since fiscal realities are generally the nemesis, they may also be the place for academic politicians to start by showing how success in human development arenas has direct economic implications through freeing up resources for other purposes. Because most prioritizing reflects an intractable bottom line, any well-wrought case will have a meaningful budgetary explanation. While decision-makers will extol human needs as being of paramount importance, the reality is that human services proposals often have softer, less measurable outcomes than, for example, miles of highway or cellblocks built. The mere perception that something is "good" is not enough as legislatures grapple with the mandate to balance budgets. The banker employs the ROI question: what is the Return On Investment? Are universities and, more specifically, human development program areas delivering ROI? Are those returns being effectively marketed to improve the credit rating for future investments? Are human development professionals effectively demonstrating that a dollar invested in their programs will multiply through positive economic gains and through diminution of health, welfare and penal system costs? The goal is to convert the perception from "Can we afford to do this?" to "We can't afford *not* to do this!"

The farmer who plants on the basis of personal affection for a crop rather than attention to market demand will not prosper. Equally, human development program administrators would do well to seed the corners of their offices with a phantom audience of taxpayers, decision-makers, and students—ubiquitous reminders of their critics, consciences and coaches. Does that silent council understand what we are doing? Are we hearing their needs? Is this serving them well? Are we delivering return on investment? Are we communicating our actions or results?" If our answer is yes, a powerful network of potential partners and advocates is being cultivated. If that network is to flourish long term, it will take constant fertilizing, replenishment, and hybridization.

Public relations are the fertilizer without which vision and substance are vacuous. The human development professions can learn a valuable lesson from the enduring strength of colleges of agriculture within land-grant universities. The early land-grant system served an agrarian society: the agricultural research, education and extension programs served the nation well and became an envied model for much of the developing world. The economic base and population demographics have changed profoundly since the first land-grant institutions dotted the prairies. And yet, agricultural units retain disproportionately strong support in the contemporary institutions. Why? First, their program emphases have changed with the times to reach new audiences in new ways. But more instructive is their prideful demonstration of return on investment, as they nurture and inform their vast network of corporate, lay, and governmental supporters about that ROI. *Substance* and *public relations*! With new audiences, new science, and complex problems spawned by families out of balance, welfare reform, a shrinking globe, changing mores, and the juxtaposition of the haves and have-nots, human development professionals have an unparalleled opportunity to similarly demonstrate their potential and their impact in competitive institutional and governmental environments. We must inform, harness, energize and empower supporters and potential partners. If we are in public institutions, and especially land-grant institutions, we need to claim a contemporary share of the historic mandate to serve society through inquiry, research, and teaching, making our knowledge base available to serve the societal and economic interests of the people. The human sciences are the agriculture of the new millennium.

Why have we not devised and marketed effective programs to overcome gigantic social problems? Bok (1990) posited that:

> Professors are often accused of being more concerned with research that will win them status in the academy than with studying firsthand the problems of poor people in urban ghettos. . . Again and again, universities have put a low priority on the very programs and initiatives that are needed most to increase productivity and competitiveness, improve the quality of government, and overcome the problems of illiteracy, miseducation and unemployment . . . [Sadly,] the vocations that attract the best students, and hence command a high priority in research universities, are rarely the careers most essential to improving competitiveness or attending to many other important social questions . . . universities are responsive, but what they respond to is what the society chooses to pay for, not what it most

> needs . . . prevailing patterns of compensation do not do a particularly good job of distributing talent in accordance with society's needs . . . Personal preferences, political pressures, and narrow time horizons all create irrational patterns of funding, such as the billions spent on finding a cure for cancer compared with the pittance made available to find effective ways of inducing people to stop smoking. (pp. 42-44)

Regrettably, the values that accord higher prestige to some professional faculties than to others, to research over teaching, and to pure research over applied research tend to become pervasive priorities in the academy. Human development professionals, as members of that academy, must first be effective advocates for change within their own houses in such areas as promotion and tenure processes: they need to challenge the conventional wisdom of the rewards system. Eugene Rice, Scholar-in-Residence with the American Association for Higher Education, explored the opportunities and pitfalls for the new American scholar-faculty "caught between the times. They are held to one set of performance criteria coming out of an earlier era and reinforced at every turn by their graduate school experience. At the same time, faculty are expected to respond to the imperatives of a vigorous change agenda aimed at improving the quality of undergraduate learning, serving the larger community, and restructuring the institution to meet rapidly shifting needs" (Rice, 1996, p. 2). Rice reviewed assumptions governing academic professionals in the rapid growth years from approximately 1957 through 1974—prevailing assumptions that shaped faculty priorities and rewards while incongruent societal needs concurrently tugged the institutions in other directions. He drew these conclusions:

1. Research is the central professional endeavor and focus of academic life.
2. Quality in the profession is maintained by peer review and professional autonomy.
3. Knowledge is pursued for its own sake.
4. The pursuit of knowledge is best organized by discipline (i.e., by discipline-based departments).
5. Reputations are established in national and international professional associations.
6. Professional rewards and mobility accrue to those who persistently accentuate their specializations.
7. The distinctive task of the academic professional is the pursuit of cognitive truth. (p. 15)

If the institutional culture is to be changed, these assumptions will have to be modified. Rice's monograph urged the academy to take a transformative approach to the way faculty work is conceived within the structure of academic careers, thus bringing greater wholeness to scholarly lives. Part of that reconceptualization would be the review of tenure requirements, certainly an area of disconnect between the perceptions of legislators and the general public about what the faculty *ought* to be doing and what they perceive faculty as actually doing—a debate made more onerous by disagreement and gradations of opinions within the academy itself. Role conflict and anxiety abound for junior faculty, caught between convictions and conventions, while abhorrence of tenure is too-often articulated by students, the general public, and especially the legislators who hold the strings of the allocation purse.

Tenure and evaluation are the genesis of the wry lamentation that "people have problems and universities have departments," the implication being that n'er shall the twain meet. The bridging of departments or disciplines seems even more chancy than the connecting of the university with the community. Interdisciplinary, multidisciplinary or work in unconventional arenas challenges established systems to a degree that junior faculty are often ill-advised to put themselves at jeopardy by such collaborative work. Sadly, this is a problem found not only in the evaluation processes undergirding tenure—decisions that theoretically should reside within the control of the faculty—but also in the machinations of budgeting and evaluation that are within the purview of administrators. Collaboration complicates bureaucratic processes. If the "new American scholar" envisioned by Rice—the scholar who will find that theoretical reflection and practice are mutually reinforcing and enriching—is going to emerge and thrive, the impetus must come from courageous leaders who will take a quantum leap in conceptualization of the roles of the university and the individual scholar and will facilitate those new roles through enlightened administrative processes.

Lombardi (1992) critiques intransigence:

> Our university subspecialties have meetings each year with sessions devoted to the topic of how to survive, prosper, or succeed under current circumstances. Each session, composed of the faithful speaking to the faithful, generally focuses on how to maximize the subspecialty's share of educational resources and opportunities by improving, enhancing, and refining that subspecialty's current agenda and improving that group's lobbying skills. . . We do not come to our meetings and advocate the dissolution of our subspecialty. We do not invite speakers who tell us we are obsolete (well, not very often and usually because we've made a mistake). We hope to leave these meetings reconfirmed that the world still loves us the way we are, that the future holds only minor modifications of our expectations, and that together with spirit we can continue much as before. . . [The result, however, of ignoring the real world of competition, changing markets and transformation, will be that] our central role in the achievement of national success will fade into an elegant, wise and irrelevant marginality. (p. 2)

PREPARING THE SOIL: "ALL POLITICS IS LOCAL"

Former House of Representatives Speaker Tip O'Neill delivered the cryptic homily that "All politics is local." Clearly, individuals being prepared for success in the public policy arena need to begin by understanding basic politics as demystified in O'Neill's comment. Success in connecting the university with the larger community begins small—person by person, at the local level, and preferably when nothing is being asked. A state agency director, who oversees a budget of nearly incomprehensible size, comments before going into crucial budget hearings, "I remind myself that we are constituents and that they represent us. I try to make their job easier by presenting our work in terms of their own legislative district rather than as a bureaucratic entitlement." She studies the special needs and services within home districts and aims to get personally acquainted with decision-makers in their own offices outside peak times. "You can learn a lot about what they think is important by seeing them in their office settings." A faculty member who has successfully secured major special state funding, serves on high level state committees, and regularly attracts powerful legislators as guest lecturers, smiles and says, "I eat a lot of barbecue. I've stuffed a lot of envelopes." She has credibility within her known political affiliation, and those across the aisle respect that, too.

The best guidance that can be given to neophytes who wish to play at the power table is to begin by participating in the political process as citizens. Learn the legislative process, model on the masters, and get to know legislators or power brokers as people. A state official, meeting with a university class as a guest professor, was astounded to find that only three of the seventy students in his class knew the name of their representative to the state legislature. Do faculty know theirs?

Political lore abounds with deals struck in between Little League innings or over hors d'oeuvres in a social setting. Legislators and other power brokers seek "face time" in the informal settings typified by church pancake suppers. An endowed professorship takes form over canapés at a country club reception. The pulse of community leaders can be taken at weekly Rotary Club luncheons. The new U.S. Representative was just the dad ladling chili at a benefit for the Cub Scouts. The most effective university politicians are those who get out of the ivory tower— often, and with relish.

A masterful academic politician describes his six-foot strategy for local politics: "I always try to let everyone within a six foot radius know something about our work," whether in social conversations, the grocery store line, or over the back fence. Observation of a corporate officer who is another consummate practical politician in a politically volatile industry, provides a lesson in building name recognition: his stash of business cards is ever-accessible, and as his cordial right hand reaches out to greet a new contact, the left hand is following through to plant a business card as a continuing reminder. Practical politics—every contact is a potential opportunity.

Even distant legislators and other key decision-makers can be localized— anointed "adopted sons/daughters" through thoughtful embracing of their knowledge. Many are pleased—indeed, flattered—to be asked to serve as guest professors either in the university setting or with students transported to the legislative environment. Take photos. Feature the occasion in newsletters. Encourage students to extend appreciation. The soil is thus prepared for both students and faculty to have future success through with decision-makers who are now friends and who have invested themselves in the educational enterprise.

Prior planning precludes poor performance. Just as the successful farmer considers crop rotations, ideal planting time, and appropriate fertilization, this prior planning on the part of human development professionals can preclude poor performance with unknown or misunderstood bureaucracies by providing key market information: What are the human needs? What are the explicit goals for me/for decision-makers? Who else cares? Who else has expertise? How can the needs and goals be collaboratively vitalized? Who are the key people who can foster the good outcomes—their special interests, their voting records, their special passions, their funding patterns? How can they be best reached? Who can best reach them? What will captivate their interest? How can initial contacts be effectively reinforced?

PLANT GOOD SEEDS

The university's greatest strength in collaborative ventures is its knowledge base, undergirded by impartial research within the spirit of academic freedom. The politically astute academician will wrestle with the ethics of when knowledge and beliefs cross the line into advocacy, and the degree of advocacy that is appropriate and acceptable.   Helping to make that determination are the quality, comprehensiveness and substance of the underlying research.

In the gardening analogy, greater vigor, color, and adaptiveness have come from hybrid seeds.   Equally, collaborations across disciplines within the university community can yield better answers to complex problems.   Best, yet, are the collaborations that engage diverse publics.

Just as seeds must be appropriate for growing conditions and climates, so initiatives to legislators and agency personnel must be tailored to special needs and interests.   Most decision-makers grapple with horrendous workloads. The goal of a proposal or of prepared testimony should be the "quick connect"—succinct, easy to read, quickly relevant. A manifesto on watch-building is an inappropriate response when someone has asked for the time. Likewise, the temptation to coat a simple statement in the idiosyncratic language of an academic discipline is a formula for failure. A legislator grunts at an obtuse tome, "What the hell does this mean?" A legislative assistant grins and shares the lingo covertly scribbled between hapless hearers during interminable, rambling testimony before committees: "MEGO," the shorthand for My Eyes Glaze Over!

Good seeds must mature within the growing season. Good proposals must fit within budgets and the timelines of legislative processes.   Understanding the realities of finances is imperative. University witnesses, effective in passionate statements of convictions, have been rendered impotent when asked about "budget notes" attached to proposed legislation—and yet, the bottom line is ultimately a crucial determinant of success or failure of many proposed measures. Showing understanding of finances and offering concrete suggestions for living within budgets are hallmarks of successful lobbyists. Because money matters are dull, sterile, and complex, they are too often neglected. "Leave that to the accountants!," we glibly say. Wrong. A recent human development master's degree recipient, interviewed two months into a state agency job, voiced her frustration: "My God, you never told me that I'd be managing a three million dollar budget. I couldn't even balance my checkbook before I took this job!" The educational enterprise failed her in an important dimension. A clear budget is propulsion for a worthy proposal: disengagement from fiscal realities can be a roadblock or a career killer.

FERTILIZE JUDICIOUSLY AND CULTIVATE WITH CARE

An experienced university president, who was legendary for his legislative prowess, credited constant vigilance for his success in maintaining effective relationships with supporting groups. Too many, he mused, emerge only to ask for something, or they believe the worthiness of an initial appeal will be self-evident. "You need to stay in the trenches," he maintained. "Don't ever sit back. Use different people in different ways to keep your needs alive before them. Try to think of fresh ways to hold their attention. Figure out how the bureaucracy works and massage it at all levels. Just when they are getting complacent, you need to come at them with an interesting new angle. They need to understand that you're not going to go away and it needs to be kind of fun."

That administrator also rued the ineptitude of many academics as negotiators. The inability to discuss to the point of finding mutual benefit has capsized many worthy ideas. "We're either too stiff-necked, self-righteous and damned inflexible or we're weak-kneed," he growled. Negotiation is a key collaborative leadership skill. A successful corporate negotiator succinctly shared his approach: First, develop a clear concept of what is wanted. Be firm on the overall goal. Write it down in concise, compelling language that others would understand: never use weak, equivocating words and never start with the "fall-back" position. Think through areas in which you could be persuaded to be flexible, considering the other person's interests, needs, and probable positions. Second, enter the process with a positive presentation of the most-desired outcomes. Make opening conditions large and opening concessions small, and give ground slowly. Try to talk less and listen more. Restate interests of the other party. Identify and stick to the key points. Stay positive, standing "for" something rather than criticizing an alternative position. Third, come to closure, parting on good terms regardless of outcome. Recognize that negotiation is a routine part of life for many decision-makers, whether formal or informal, and the person who comes either to the table or into a chance interaction with clear goals and good facts will be more likely to succeed.

SHARING THE WORK: THE CASE FOR COLLABORATION

At a conference on partnerships between the university and state government, an economist set the theme as follows: "A partnership is an association of two or more parties who enter into an agreement from which they can each benefit or lose." Societal problems are inherently interdisciplinary and are often best managed by partners with differing expertise. Corporate management theory acknowledges this as companies move from hierarchical structures to lattices, webs or grids.

Collaborative leadership, however, poses special challenges to academics accustomed to functioning as "authority figures," as well as to those who exercise control within other bureaucratic settings. Coming together requires respect for diversity and willingness to function in unfamiliar contexts. Effective communication is imperative. Teams need to be built with a clear sense of goals, potential resources, and empowerment to make decisions and solve problems through consensus or negotiation.

All of these are skills that should be inherent in human development programs. Human development professionals should feel sustained at any negotiating table or in proposing partnerships because we are inherently strong partners for these reasons:

First, we have a *socially relevant knowledge base*—the skills and knowledge to improve the economic, environmental, social, psychological, aesthetic and physiological aspects of the lives of the family, community and marketplace. Our work has an unabashed *values* dimension. From the vision of founders to the present, our education has an *activist core* based on knowledge and ethics. We are *scholars of the family and community*, clearly the primary social and economic units in America and thus important to other professions and institutions. Power brokers respond to our expertise when explained in terms of their own life experiences, needs and business goals. Corporate America has family concerns. It markets to a changing society. Its employees come from families under stress, juggling jobs, schedules, parenting, and resources. Stability and mores in the family structure are at the root of the preponderance of problems confronting government.

Second, we offer long standing *networks working with families* through Cooperative Extension programs and agencies serving families.

Third, the predominantly *female demographics* in many human development professions can be an asset in requesting a place at discussion tables. Although 52% of the population is female, decisions are too often made by bodies that are open to criticism because of their lopsided representation.

Fourth, human development disciplines offer a *holistic, lifespan, developmental perspective* that spans the hierarchy of human needs from most basic to self-actualizing and across the entire span of ages and experiences. Our understanding of the interconnectedness of needs at various stages can span narrower interest groups.

Fifth, we *staff the economy* in some of the nation's major industries and especially in the burgeoning service sector.

In short, we are good partners ourselves. But if human development professionals are to be effective in offering significant societal service, garnering respect, receiving fiscal and psychic support, and building the most effective vision and knowledge for the century ahead, we also need to augment the advocacy strength of our ranks with others. There is strength in numbers and in unity. Who can join us?

First, we can find superb potential partners in *unexpected units within our own institutions*—perhaps in disciplines quite different from our own. An economist, a physician, a lawyer, or an engineer might well lend an unexpected and compelling dimension to a proposal. And, just as parents beam when the children are playing nicely together, institutional administrators express pride in cross-disciplinary collaboration. Of course territoriality exists and to suggest otherwise would be mindlessly naïve. But, valued partnerships can and should evolve if we focus on a need and how to meet it rather than on self interest. Remember that six foot rule? Can others in our own institutions clearly articulate our potential contributions to partnerships?

Campus administrators should also be partners. Our relevancy can make the institution look good, while they can help us by their connections and support. They need a sense of ownership of our achievements. Give them the working phrases to easily describe what we do. Seek counsel. Assertively expect that the agenda of the applied social sciences will move to the fore in institutional support, just as a small Soviet beeping ball in space catapulted mathematics and science decades ago. Point out that the beeping balls that are threatening daily quality of life in this nation are a consequence of earlier neglect in funding and other priorities. Money for social pathologies siphons money for education: thus, they have a vested interest in our success.

Students are magnificent partners. Informed and enthusiastic students can outdo their elders in areas of recruitment, activism, and legislative impact. They can be effusive, articulate, and prescriptive. They and their parents live in legislative districts where their viewpoints carry clout. Notable successes occur when appropriately prepared students interact with legislative or corporate officials in symposia, meal functions, hearings, and in office calls. Students can rapidly evolve to sophisticated lobbyists if part of the college culture includes factual discussion of public policy issues.

The current impetus to include service as an integral part of the academic curriculum augurs well for informed students who progress to enlightened and competent citizenry. "Service learning" is moving from isolated experimental programs to mainstream programs in many institutions. Work with community agencies and legislative internships plunges students into real life experiences that achieve greatest effectiveness under close mentorship that links hands-on experiences with the intellectual base. Alexander Astin described preliminary findings from the work of the Higher Education Research Institute relating to the benefits to college students involved in volunteer service and service learning. Thirty-four outcome measures falling in the areas of civic responsibility, academic development, and life skills development all appear to be positively affected by undergraduate experiences in volunteer experience. Service learning is also linked to long-term outcomes that relate to enlightened civic participation (Astin, 1996).

Alumni, too, are strong allies, and yet many units have not harnessed their power. Small groups of articulate alumni can accomplish feats that faculty and administrators cannot. Legislative networks of alumni, cultivated and informed over time, can provide matchless local interest, connections, and impetus.

Powerful allies are *business and professional advisory boards* for professional programs. Many colleges have alumni boards or boards of visitors. However, constellations of high level people from business, government, and agencies who are brought together to guide the development of single departments are invaluable resources because they daily deal with problems that are real, complex and intractable. They are relevance personified. Most successful people have a desire to give something back and will take a proprietorial interest in programs, becoming dynamic advocates. Most have, as a hallmark of success, developed networks that lead to centers of power.

The *media*, occasionally a nemesis, can also be a partner. News organizations are criticized for focusing only on pathologies, and some would suggest that people are more interested in problems than good news. Willingness to work with reporters to vitalize and communicate success stories is an important complement to professional skills. A favorable story in the local press can be a fog-cutter in getting the attention of others.

HARVEST THE RESULTS

Build on strengths. Savor successes. Correct weaknesses. Take the long view. Have a tolerance for delayed gratification. Platitudes? No. Human needs develop over time. It takes time to harness the forces to effectively address problems and opportunities. It takes time to establish credibility and build trust. Legislative and social agendas do not turn on tenure clocks. Agendas do not necessarily prevail just because we are personally convinced of their worth. The ability to self-critique, possibly regroup, and move on is an imperative skill in building partnerships between the university and the larger community.

The Policymakers' Program of the Danforth Foundation found that states (substitute "human development professionals") that have been *most successful* in effecting better results for children and families have advocates within the legislative and executive branches of government and agency heads who demonstrate strong collaborative leadership. Progress in the human services relates to a supportive governor, bipartisanship, strong collaborative leadership among education, human services, and health agencies, and a community-based approach (Parsons & Brumbaugh, 1996).

On the other hand, the Danforth-sponsored discussions found that success was impaired by political changes, turf protecting, insufficient attention to the building of local momentum, and lack of team leadership. The message from professionals whose jobs are at the apex of visibility within their states is straight-forward: political activism and good causes alone are vacuous without solid skills and careful collaboration. Their recurring themes were: *needs-based, locally-oriented, collaboratively coordinated and implemented, accountability for ROI (return on investment), realistic understanding of available resources.* With this approach, good seed is sown on fertile soil that has been well cultivated, yielding a probability of good harvests.

EXPRESS APPRECIATION

The final step in any collaborative enterprise is the savoring of successes and the expression of appreciation. Legislators reflect that they hear the passion of pleas, but all too rarely are apprised of results or thanked for their assistance. The teacher who receives a letter from an appreciative graduate savors and rereads and perhaps saves it—highlighting the rarity of the experience. The act of expressing

70

Social Change, Public Policy, and Community Collaborations: Training
Human Development Professionals for the Twenty-First Century

appreciation and generously giving credit prepares the seedbed for future collaborations.

SUMMARY

The analogy of a politically pragmatic approach to building community relationships to enlightened farming practices begins with the legitimization of getting in tune with the earth and the market, which requires exiting the ivory tower. This is an overdue process, weighted by history, fraught with conditions out of one's direct control, and requiring careful study of market needs and trends. However, success can yield great benefits to the larger society as well as to the academic milieu. The challenge is to create a well-wrought process that effectively analyzes and demonstrates return on investment. Obstacles to be overcome include antiquated promotion and tenure evaluative procedures and the inflexibility of bureaucratic systems in accommodating to new forms of collaboration and scholarship. Basic to success are the planning and careful analysis of the seedbed in which ideas will be planted, well-chosen and well-executed initiatives, and hands-on cultivation and nurturing of decision-makers and collaborators through proven techniques of public relations and negotiation. Partnerships that enhance potential for successful outcomes are examined, with emphasis on the special strengths of the human development disciplines. Last, the harvesting of results is accompanied by planning for the future and the expression of appreciation to those who contributed to success.

REFERENCES

Astin, A. (1996, March/April). The role of service in higher education. *About Campus*, 14-19.

Bok, D. (1990). *Universities and the future of America*. Durham and London: Duke University Press.

Goldman, J. J. (1990, August 7). Universities rated 'F' for inability to help solve society's problems. *Los Angeles Times*, A5.

Keller, R. (1997, February 18). Senator throws prison challenge at UM. *Columbia Daily Tribune*, 1.

Lombardi, J. V. (1992). *Who are we and where are we going?* Presentation at the National Land Grant Lay Leaders Seminar. Washington, DC: National Association of State Universities and Land Grant Colleges.

Parsons, B. A. & Brumbaugh, S. (1996). How leadership and policy development are affecting practice through education and human services collaborations. *Policymakers' Program Evaluation Report, Year 4*. Danforth Foundation Report.

Rice, E. (1996). Making a place for the new American scholar. *New Pathways Working Paper Series, Inquiry #1*. Washington, DC: American Association for Higher Education.

The Children, Youth, and Family Consortium: A University of Minnesota/Community Partnership[1]

Martha Farrell Erickson and Richard A. Weinberg
University of Minnesota

In a time of careful scrutiny of public spending, public universities—which absorb a large portion of state educational resources—are challenged more than ever before to be accountable. Often driven by a land-grant mission, universities are under the microscope to demonstrate efficient deployment of resources in addressing educational needs and applying research to practice for the benefit of their constituents. The ivory tower is tilting under a vigorous press to eliminate program redundancy, pursue new target audiences, widen the scope of extension teaching and adult education, retool professionals for the changing job market, and promote outreach activities that address community needs (Weinberg, Fishhaut, Moore & Plaisance, 1990).

Institutions of higher learning also feel the pressures that stem from a society in turmoil. Children, youth, and families in Minnesota, not unlike those in other states, face enormous challenges at the brink of the twenty-first century: economic distress, isolation, violence, substance abuse, teenage pregnancy, inadequate health care, and strained educational and human-service systems. These problems will not wait. The price of delay is too heavy by any measure, from the unforgivable loss of human capital to the staggering costs of future remediation. The University of Minnesota, with its wealth of knowledge and resources on children, youth, and family issues, has a strong obligation to understand and respond to these needs and challenges.

It is in this context that the Children, Youth, and Family Consortium at the University of Minnesota was created. Founded in November 1991, the Consortium reflects the growing commitment of faculty and community professionals to nurture a far-reaching, cross-disciplinary, community-based effort to address the pressing needs of Minnesota's children, youth, and families. Although still (and ever) evolving, the Consortium provides a model of a public university as a vital and dynamic force for the well-being of children and the strengthening of families and communities. And, on a broader level, it is an example of systems change that could apply to other topics and disciplines as well.

In this chapter we present a case study of the Consortium, an innovation that has evolved in the current sociopolitical climate but that is rooted in the unique traditions and context of the University of Minnesota. The growth and direction of the Consortium have been guided by particular circumstances and events unique to the setting and its stakeholders. Here we highlight the early history of the Consortium, set out the guiding principles and mission that fuel its development, summarize the first five years of its activities, and discuss some of the hurdles that have been confronted during this formative period.

SETTING THE STAGE

As a land-grant institution, the University of Minnesota already had established by 1991 a legacy of cooperation in addressing children, youth, and family issues by connecting related activities within the University and forging links with the community. These included:

- cross-departmental centers, institutes, and an extension service with particular goals and constituents in mind, funded through a wide range of internal and external sources;
- professional training programs with multidisciplinary foci;
- collaboratives of faculty and community people for the pursuit of research, teaching, and service-outreach;
- formal and informal communication networks among University and community groups.

Furthermore, the University had earned a solid reputation, within the state of Minnesota and nationally, for top-quality research and teaching in child and family-focused fields.

These achievements notwithstanding, our efforts seldom had been coordinated or leveraged in a way to maximize their impact. As a fundamental example, the University had no inventory of its own personnel and research and outreach activities in the area of children, youth, and families—a serious obstacle to internal and external synergism. We were driven by an appreciation of the problems and ideas about how to solve some of them. Collectively, we were aware that we know much more than we used or applied; we had to begin to translate that interdisciplinary knowledge into action that would have true impact on the lives of Minnesota's children and youth.

We were guided also by the fact that a university can do little in isolation. The best hope for impact is through partnership with individuals and agencies in the community who know the crises first-hand and who may be piloting innovation. Collaborative effort is no longer a choice—it is a necessity. This consortium, unlike some past efforts, could be neither paternalistic nor unilateral. A clear acknowledgment of the authority of both the University and the community would be integral to planning and guiding the Consortium's development. It would be imperative that both worlds be fully invested in this effort to ensure its success.

We were also aware that we had an unprecedented window of opportunity to take advantage of heightened public interest and more open pockets in the area of children, youth, and families. But the window would not be open forever. As Anthony Downs (1972) wisely cautioned over twenty years ago, public attention rarely focuses on one domestic issue for very long, even if it involves a problem of crucial importance to society. Typically, problems leap into prominence, remain there for a short time, then—even though unresolved—fade from the center of attention. Because that kind of focused public scrutiny and the political pressure it can engender are essential to the implementation of change, the climate of concern about children, youth, and families made the timing for a University-community consortium ideal.

THE RETREAT

A concerned and impassioned group of faculty and community representatives set the stage for this initiative, determined not to do simply a better job at what they had already undertaken but to try a new and different strategy. Building on the legacy of cooperation between town and gown established over time, a steering committee hosted a one-and-a-half-day planning retreat in late 1990, with thirty-nine faculty and eleven community representatives participating. In early fall, Twin Cities campus deans and chancellors on other campuses had been asked to nominate University candidates; steering committee members had recommended community candidates. Participants were selected on the basis of fair and balanced representation of gender, area of expertise, and ethnicity.

A set of broad questions guided the agenda for the retreat:

- Have the University's research, teaching, and service activities to date really made a difference in the lives of Minnesota's children, youth, and families?
- Are we effectively marshaling the considerable expertise and resources of the University and community in setting agendas for meeting the needs of those populations?
- Have we been proactive as well as reactive in guiding the course of our efforts?
- Do we even know the key players within the University and community, and do we create sufficient opportunities for them to share perspectives and to participate in joint ventures?

GUIDING PRINCIPLES AND MISSION

The outcome of this highly productive retreat was a set of guiding principles to provide direction to the development of the consortium:

8. The press for an all-University/community collaboration to improve the lives of Minnesota's children, youth, and families originates in a social/economic/political Zeitgeist that has raised our collective consciousness, irrespective of our individual disciplines.
9. There is a great need for a forum that links University and community personnel interested in children, youth, and families. Such a forum would create a much-needed symbiosis, nourishing the work of community practitioners and enriching the work of academic researchers.
10. The current state of tension between the University and community agencies cannot be ignored. Problems seem to stem from the two parties' diverging missions and culture types: The University is a deliberative culture where knowledge is generated and disseminated, while community agencies are action-oriented providers of direct service. To be effective, this consortium must be grounded in the principle of reciprocity and mutual respect between the community and University.
11. The consortium idea reflects the need for an organizing/coordinating mechanism among the many University units active in the area of children, youth, and families. It does not imply the need for another such unit. The consortium is best thought of as a process not a structure. (Note that once established, the consortium subsequently was described by some as an "attitude" or even an "essence.") A consortium should create a culture, an environment that empowers faculty and community professionals to work more effectively on behalf of children, youth, and families.
12. This consortium should attempt to develop a matrix of concerns about children, youth, and families throughout the state. Information sharing and synergism should be encouraged not only at the intra-University level, but also at community and state levels as well, so that all those working for

improvements understand each other's programs and are supportive whenever possible. For example, at the University level, this would mean connecting the child health activities of the pediatrics department with research and policy initiatives in the Institute of Child Development, the Department of Family Social Science, and the Institute on Community Integration, and linking all those units to the dissemination efforts of others such as the Minnesota Extension Service and the Center for Early Education and Development.

13. The intent of this consortium is to be inclusive rather than exclusive. Membership should be open to all individuals and agencies with interest in the well-being of children, youth, and families. The strength of this network will depend on the multidisciplinary, intersectional (community, University), ethnically diverse character of its membership.

14. This effort to launch a cooperative, multidisciplinary attack on a range of critical societal problems is congruent with the University's growing emphases on maximizing efficiency, cross-departmental planning, and responsiveness to state needs. Our proposal seeks to better coordinate existing resources for optimal effectiveness.

In November 1991, the Consortium turned on its lights and telephones and set out to pursue its mission, as defined at the planning retreat:

> . . . to bring together the varied competencies of the University of Minnesota and the vital resources of Minnesota's communities to enhance the ability of individuals and organizations to address critical health, education, and social policy concerns in ways that improve the well-being of Minnesota children, youth, and families.

THE START-UP

Guided by a motivational statement made at the end of the planning Retreat to "Get going fast! Don't lose the momentum!" we moved into action to establish a structure and begin our work:

1. We expanded the existing faculty Steering Committee to include community representation from greater Minnesota as well as the metropolitan Twin Cities area. The committee would report to the president of the University.

2. We established a Consortium office, separate from any existing University unit, and easily accessible for individuals from the community.

3. We established a nominal staff structure to include a part-time coordinator (subsequently upgraded to director), secretary, and other staff to oversee and coordinate Consortium activities and to staff the Steering Committee.

4. We actively promoted Consortium participation for University and community professionals interested in the well-being of children, youth, and families (CYF).

5. We established regular meetings of the expanded Steering Committee and more frequent meetings of the Executive Committee, a subset of the larger group committed to working closely with staff until the Consortium was solidly established.

6. We also established work groups to bring people together face-to-face on a regular basis to pursue common goals that enhance their own work and serve the needs of young people, families, and the professionals who work

with them. Each work group was co-facilitated by a University person and a professional from the community at large. The groups functioned in an autonomous, self-directed way with support and assistance from Consortium staff. Groups were expected to form, transform, end, and reform as necessary, remaining dynamic and responsive to the changing needs and challenges around CYF issues.

FIVE YEARS LATER: WHERE IS THE CONSORTIUM TODAY?

Since its inception, the Consortium has been the catalyst for exciting collaboration across a wide range of CYF issues. Through symposia, publications, ongoing work groups, innovative use of technology, partnership with grassroots community initiatives, and collaborative grant seeking, the Consortium has taken its place as a central agent in bringing about meaningful change for Minnesota communities and ensuring that the University of Minnesota is an active partner in the process. More than twenty-three academic departments and units, twenty University centers, and the Minnesota Extension Service are joining efforts and pooling resources. The Consortium Advisory Council (formerly Steering Committee) is more broadly representative—and more actively involved in Consortium activities—than ever before. In addition, a Deans Policy Group meets quarterly to ensure investment and participation across all relevant colleges.

Most importantly, the Consortium is fulfilling a moral and ethical responsibility to "give away" information and put our knowledge to work on behalf of children, youth, and their families. Furthermore, we are listening constantly to the larger Minnesota community (and, increasingly, communities across the nation), working to see that our teaching and research agendas are informed by community wisdom.

The accomplishments and ongoing activities of the Consortium can be profiled best according to the three facets of the University's land-grant mission: instruction, research, and outreach. (Note that in reality those three facets are intricately interwoven and activities rarely fall solely into one category.) While special events and short-term projects (e.g., conferences and symposia, an annual holiday book drive [Food for Thought], and public-awareness campaigns) should be part of the Consortium in order to ensure visibility and bring people together around current issues, our primary intent is to focus our energy and resources toward systems change.

INSTRUCTION

From the early planning stages of the Consortium, we have heard from community representatives that universities send too many professionals into the field who are not prepared to function in a cross-disciplinary world. Although we have given lip service to ideas of cross-disciplinary education and we recognize that the situations facing professionals demand it, educational practice has continued to be centered largely within isolated departments and disciplines. Furthermore, CYF issues demand that all citizens—not only the usual CYF professionals—share responsibility for the well-being of children and families. Yet, university programs often do little to prepare students to assume that responsibility, nor do we prepare our CYF professional students to work effectively with the broader citizenry in addressing CYF needs. No longer can disciplines educate in parallel with other disciplines on interrelated issues. In addition, we cannot afford to ignore broad community expertise in developing practitioners and community leaders into the year 2000.

With this in mind, the Consortium has been the nexus of planning for several major cross-disciplinary instructional initiatives:

- A series of noncredit seminars on raising safe, healthy children, offered through the Compleat Scholar program for University employees and students. The seminars have been facilitated jointly by University and community experts.
- A descriptive directory of CYF course offerings at the University, available as a part of the Consortium Electronic Clearinghouse (described in a later section of this chapter).
- Development of a new extension program to educate and certify CYF workers, in partnership with Early Childhood Studies through Continuing Education and Extension.
- Implementation of interdisciplinary training in adolescent development as a part of the Adolescent Health Partnership. (This partnership, which also encompasses research and outreach activities, is described in some detail in Weinberg & Erickson, 1996.)
- Internships for graduate and undergraduate students providing unique cross-disciplinary, community-linked, learning opportunities.
- An initiative funded by the Minnesota Higher Education Coordinating Board that focuses on transdisciplinary professional education in service to children and families. This project includes:
  1. development of an all-university graduate-level seminar designed to enhance the collaborative professional competencies of students from diverse disciplines;
  2. establishment of a work group aimed at reconciling the unique, narrow, specialized credentialing requirements of individual disciplines by examining barriers to licensing and credentialing of professionals, and identifying next steps toward the goal of inclusive, transdisciplinary educational and credentialing requirements.
- Establishment of a University-funded interdepartmental task force to improve coordination of course offerings and training among various University units providing education in mental-health practice.

RESEARCH

In a time of limited resources, departments and units with similar purposes too often compete against each other rather than join forces. The Consortium is playing a central role, both within the University and between the University and the community at large, in organizing people around ideas, leveraging resources, and aggressively pursuing new outside funding for research that addresses real community issues. Much of the Consortium's effort in the area of research is driven by what the community tells us they want from the University: Research that addresses their pressing issues, with findings shared promptly in a way that is understandable and useful. Throughout the community we also hear a cry for the University to ensure that its students in CYF programs enter the field of practice with a solid understanding of how to conduct evaluation research. And, facing increasing pressure from funders and the general public to demonstrate the effectiveness of their programs, CYF service providers are calling on the University to provide ongoing training and technical assistance to professionals already in the field. In the domain of research our accomplishments thus far include:

- Partnership in Kids Count with the Children's Defense Fund, Congregations Concerned for Children, and the Minnesota Extension

Service. Data from Kids Count are available on the Consortium Electronic Clearinghouse to facilitate research on the status and well-being of children throughout Minnesota.

- Identification of factors that facilitate or hinder University-community collaborative research, and successful efforts to eliminate some of the barriers to such collaboration (e.g., library privileges for community research collaborators).
- A major conference on evaluating CYF programs, jointly sponsored with the Minnesota Chapter of the American Evaluation Association, followed by an ongoing series of skill-building workshops on evaluation strategies.
- Creation of an evaluation research section on the Consortium Electronic Clearinghouse (described later).
- Formation of the Adolescent Health Partnership (mentioned earlier under "Instruction"), which designs and implements creative, interdisciplinary evaluations of community interventions and proposed youth policies at the national, state, and local level.
- Matching faculty and graduate students for paid or volunteer consultation on evaluation initiatives at community agencies (e.g., Washburn Child Guidance Center, St. David's School, and the Hennepin County Children's Mental Health Initiative).
- Coordination of a major evaluation and research project with the Institute on Community Integration as part of the Minneapolis Area Learning Readiness Initiative.
- For the U.S. Department of Health and Human Services, preparation of a synthesis of research on fathering, leading to the development of a theoretical framework to guide DHHS in their efforts to encourage father involvement and responsibility. This synthesis is informed by our work with father support leaders in Minnesota, and by a national network of practitioners and researchers working on fatherhood issues. The work is an outgrowth of our involvement in Vice President Gore's annual family policy conferences, as described below under our outreach activities.
- Participation in a national network of researchers coordinated by the National Center on Fathers and Families at the University of Pennsylvania, with a goal of creating an extensive research library on fathering and identifying new areas of practical fatherhood research to pursue collaboratively.

OUTREACH

At a time when relations between the University and Minnesota's communities often have been strained at best, the outreach efforts of the Consortium are especially critical. In close partnership with the Minnesota Extension Service, the Consortium makes the University more user-friendly and ensures that the vital knowledge of the University is put to work effectively in communities around the state. We view this as the area in which we have brought about the greatest change in the five years since the Consortium was founded.

In a relatively brief time we have achieved high visibility in the community. We have established a public identity as a "place" where people can connect with others and can find access to resources about children, youth, and families. We have accomplished that largely by reaching out to community organizations as they plan their own efforts to address the needs of children and families. We have demonstrated that we are not trying to claim credit or ownership, but to support and facilitate, helping to make sure that efforts are grounded in the latest research on what really matters for young people and their families. Outreach activities have included:

- Publishing a quarterly newsletter, "Community Connections," that goes to over 9,000 people and is designed to present information on CYF programs around the state and to enhance connections and collaborations among people within the University and throughout Minnesota. The newsletter includes substantive articles about work in progress; a calendar of relevant University and community events; summaries of Consortium work-group activities; and a "Connection Corner" column that allows readers to seek program volunteers, information and materials, or colleagues with whom to collaborate or exchange information.
- Coordinating the first Minnesota Children's Summit, which brought together 250 leaders from throughout the state for a research-based, action-oriented dialogue about what we know about supporting the healthy development of children, youth, and families.
- Producing a forty-minute video of highlights of the Children's Summit, with accompanying study guide, to serve as a springboard for discussion and action at the local community level.
- Developing and disseminating a set of guiding principles to help parents, professionals, and policy makers determine if their decisions take into account the basic needs and rights of children.
- Supporting grassroots public awareness and community education initiatives, including "The Village Project" in Washington County, the "Kids—Handle with Care" project in Goodhue County, and the statewide "Turn Off the Violence" campaign.
- Linking the University with broad community initiatives, including the Children's Initiative, Minneapolis's Neighborhood Revitalization Project, the United Way's Vision Councils, "Success by Six," and St. Paul's Safe Cities Initiative.
- Working with various organizations around the state to develop a coordinated effort to provide parenting education and support for parents of school-age and adolescent children. As one major step in this initiative, we have implemented the Homework Project, which documents existing resources for parents of children of all ages and promotes these resources through a printed catalogue and an on-line directory.
- Coordinating the "University in the Community Project," which brought University faculty and administrators face-to-face with people in diverse communities around the state to listen to community concerns and let citizens know how the University can be a resource to them.
- Implementing the "Community Connectors Institute," funded by the McKnight Foundation, which brought together a diverse, interdisciplinary cohort group from each of three Minnesota communities for an innovative process of education and problem solving.
- "Giving away" information to the media, including a parenting column in small-town newspapers throughout the Upper Midwest, a weekly radio feature on forty Minnesota stations, and a weekly television feature on the Twin Cities NBC affiliate.
- In partnership with the Star Tribune newspaper and WCCO-TV, presenting a series of four photojournalistic reports entitled "Seeds of Violence or Seeds of Promise." These clear and compelling reports, and the accompanying TV news features and newspaper commentaries, are designed to educate the public about risk and resiliency in children, to let

people know how they can make a difference in the lives of children in their families and communities, and to point them to helpful resources.

- Promoting the "Safe Team" campaign, a joint effort with KMSP-TV and the Minnesota Department of Children, Families, and Learning, to teach and encourage nonviolent conflict resolution among school age children.
- Building relationships beyond Minnesota, working with colleague organizations such as the Applied Developmental Science Consortium (which includes Michigan State University, Fordham University, Pennsylvania State University, University of Nebraska, and Johns Hopkins University). This group of universities, primarily land-grant institutions, has been exploring ways to collaborate in the translation and application of developmental knowledge to societal problems.
- Hosting "Family Re-Union," an annual national conference moderated in Nashville by Vice President and Mrs. Gore, bringing together each year one thousand researchers, program leaders, and policy makers to explore critical issues in family policy. These conferences have addressed "The Role of Men in Children's Lives," "Media and the Family," and "Work and Family," and have informed ongoing action plans both in Minnesota and on a national level.
- As an outgrowth of Family Re-Union III, coordinating the development of "Father to Father," a national movement to "Unite fathers for their children and mobilize communities for fathers and their families." As a part of this national effort, we also have worked with Minnesota leaders in the father support movement to sustain an ongoing practitioner network and stimulate new community support for Minnesota fathers.
- As an outgrowth of Family Re-Union IV (Media and the Family), working with the Office of the Attorney General of Minnesota and the Minnesota Medical Association to lead a three-pronged campaign to promote more positive use of media for the sake of children. The three strands of activity include media literacy training for parents and classroom teachers; a corporate responsibility campaign aimed at advertisers and leaders in the media industry; and the grassroots "Turn Off the Violence" campaign.
- Launching "Seeds of Promise," a University-wide outreach effort to address the needs of Twin Cities urban children and youth. Organized around the conceptual framework of the importance of caring adults in the life of a child, this new initiative integrates research, teaching, and service activities with a focus on the urban communities in which the University of Minnesota is located. We are reaching beyond the usual CYF departments and units at the University to include students, faculty, staff, and alumni from all departments in this major effort to respond to the Twin Cities communities' call for us to: 1) Make our research relevant and useful in addressing the needs of urban youth; 2) help evaluate the effectiveness of programs that aim to strengthen the connection of children and youth with caring adults in their families and neighborhoods; and 3) "roll up our sleeves" and work alongside other community members in reaching out to urban children and families. With a small planning grant from the Danforth Foundation, this initiative is just getting underway, but already it has sparked the interest and commitment of many University citizens outside the usual CYF circle.

THE CONSORTIUM ELECTRONIC CLEARINGHOUSE (CEC)

Certainly, there are many Consortium activities that serve purposes across all three functions of the land-grant mission. One such bridging activity that deserves special recognition is CEC (we say "seek"). The original plan for the Consortium included a goal of creating an extended "rolodex" of people and programs that deal with CYF issues. This was one of the first activities that we pursued when the Consortium offices opened. We soon recognized the need—and the potential—for something much larger than the "rolodex" as originally envisioned. We discovered that within the University was the technology and the know-how to create a user-friendly system by which professionals and the general public might acquire current information about children, youth, and families. Thus, in partnership with the Minnesota Extension Service, we began to develop CEC, an Internet web site, which includes the original concept and much more.

We also discovered that many organizations within and outside of the university had similar visions, but none had taken significant action in realizing their plans. Consequently, we played a catalytic role in bringing together representatives of those groups and figuring out how we could achieve our goals efficiently and effectively together. As a result, CEC now houses data from Kids Count (a Children's Defense Fund/Congregations Concerned for Children project), serves as the gateway of information exchange on adoption issues (AdoptInfo), facilitates a wide range of work on fathering (FatherNet, created in conjunction with Family Re-Union III), and links users to multiple resources on media and the family (MediaForum, created as an outgrowth of Family Re-Union IV). Beyond these and other specialized resource centers, CEC manages and updates a wide range of general informational resources on a variety of CYF topics, including many newsletters and small publications that otherwise would reach very limited audiences. And, in cases where quality resources already exist on-line, CEC points to those sites to ensure a "seamless" experience for the user.

Consortium staff often make presentations about CEC at professional conferences and community events, and they provide free or low-cost training tailored to the needs of specific agencies so that professionals and lay people can take advantage of this rich electronic resource. CEC is the major tool by which we facilitate information exchange and connect people with needed resources. Thanks to a remarkably dedicated CEC advisory board, whose community and University members bring strong content knowledge, technical expertise, and an understanding of information management, CEC is perhaps our clearest example of a real synergistic partnership. To date, thousands of individuals have accessed CEC. Our intent is to continue to harness resources to create real order and value on the electronic information highway, for the well-being of children, youth, and families.

BARRIERS TO CHANGE

In five years the Consortium has made substantial progress in accomplishing its mission, but we know that we still have a long way to go. In particular, we are working hard to:

1. increase the level of involvement and commitment of stakeholders within the University such that the synergy made possible through the Consortium becomes a way of doing daily business;
2. broaden the base of involvement within the University, reaching beyond the usual CYF units to engage the entire University community in working

toward the well-being of Minnesota's citizens ("Seeds of Promise" is a significant step toward this goal);

3. increase and strengthen our connections with professionals from outside the metropolitan area to ensure that the Consortium works for the benefit of all Minnesotans;

4. reach out to other Minnesota institutions of higher learning to build a rich network of cross-disciplinary educational experiences for pre- and in-service professionals in CYF-related fields.

As with all of our Consortium activities, the results of these efforts will be evaluated in terms of their "value-added" uniqueness and centrality to the mission of a land-grant university.

We would be remiss if we created a Pollyanna image that there have been no obstacles to establishing the Consortium. Resistance to change is not uncommon where traditional paradigms and the status quo are challenged. Our experience is not unlike what others have encountered in attempting to modify the way the academy goes about its work (e.g., Lawson & Hooper-Briar, 1994). The most critical barriers that the Consortium continually confronts include:

Distrust of the University

The community often looks on the University with considerable mistrust. A number of explanations seem to account for this climate of tension:

- *Perceptions of University arrogance, egocentrism, and paternalism*: "The University takes, but it doesn't give back." The University often uses community sources for research but seldom shares the results of that research with these sources.
- *Difficult access*: The complex structure of the University is confusing to outsiders; physical barriers to visitors, especially parking, are often insurmountable.
- *Poor communication*: The University's goals and purposes in research are not clearly explained to community collaborators.
- *Lack of acknowledgment that the University and the community are different cultures exploring unique missions*: The University generates and disseminates knowledge and often addresses long-term solutions to long-term problems, but the community provides direct service and often must provide prompt intervention with short-term results.

The University Reward System

The University historically appears to penalize faculty who excel in service and community-outreach activities by not weighting those accomplishments equally with research and teaching in promotion and tenure decisions, salary merit increases, and other aspects of faculty career development. Furthermore, interdepartmental collaboration appears to be a disincentive when an individual faculty member's "independent" scholarly contributions are reviewed. This model must be modified if effective cooperative ventures are to be supported.

Turfdom Among the Disciplines

Unfortunately, intellectual and professional "territorialism" pervade the academy and the professions that serve the needs of children, youth, and families (Lerner & Fisher, 1994). We have recognized that the disciplines that typically have defined practice in the area of CYF do not necessarily provide the most effective paradigm for education and service in today's world. New ways of preparing and supporting professionals who serve those populations must be explored. The time is right to identify the common knowledge and competencies that cut across disciplines, to tear down (or at least cut windows in) the walls that separate disciplines, and to educate and serve in a way that is driven by the needs of children, youth, and families rather than by departmental or disciplinary labels.

Funding Issues

The work of the Consortium is not peripheral, not some "extra" that has been added onto a core of traditional activities pursued by the University. And yet initially, in terms of financial support, the Consortium was treated in some ways as an "extra." Operating on a bare-bones budget, the Consortium relied largely on the goodwill of staff and committee members who worked well beyond compensation. We knew that to fulfill our vision and mission, we must have a more realistic, stable financial base. Fortunately, the passion underlying the development of the Consortium was shared by members of central administration who shape the University's budget. But ironically, at a time of retrenchment and reallocation, funds provided to the Consortium are likely drawn away from the constituent departments and units the Consortium hopes to bring together. The generation of external support from foundations and other funding sources requires that the Consortium have a secure and adequate institutional funding base. While our general operational funding is more generous and stable than it was initially, we still sustain our momentum with more heart than dollars.

CONCLUSIONS: ACHIEVING THE VISION

We believe the Children Youth, and Family Consortium at the University of Minnesota is: 1) an effective prototype of how land-grant institutions can create linkages among disciplines to accomplish shared goals for meeting the needs of our nation's children, youth, families, and communities, and 2) a dynamic, reciprocal model for connecting a university with its communities.

As universities reassess, redefine, and restructure, the Consortium provides an innovative and practical example of systems change for community good. We hope that the financial, psychological, and emotional resources will continue to be sufficient to sustain and nurture this exciting collaboration and outreach enterprise.

NOTE

1. This chapter is reprinted from the book, *University-community collaborations for the twenty-first century: Outreach scholarship for youth and families*, edited by R. M. Lerner & L. A. K. Simon, 1998, Garland Publishing, New York, NY. For additional information about the Children, Youth, and Family Consortium, please write to University of Minnesota, 12 McNeal Hall, 1985 Buford Avenue, St. Paul, MN 55108.

REFERENCES

Downs, A. (1972). Up and down with ecology: The issue-attention cycle. *The Public Interest, 29*, 38-50.

Lawson, H. A. & Hooper-Briar, K. (1994). *Expanding partnerships: Involving colleges and universities in interprofessional collaboration and service integration.* Oxford, OH: The Danforth Foundation and the Institute for Educational Renewal at Miami University.

Lerner, R. M., & Fisher, C. M. (1994). From applied developmental psychology to applied developmental services: Community coalition and collaborative careers. In C. B. Fisher & R. M. Lerner, (Eds.), *Applied Developmental Psychology.* New York: McGraw-Hill.

Weinberg, R. A. & Erickson, M. F. (1996). Minnesota's children, youth, and family consortium: A university-community collaboration. *Journal of Research on Adolescence, 61*, 37-53.

Weinberg, R. A., Fishhaut, E. H., Moore, S. G., & Plaisance, C. (1990, December). The Center for Early Education and Development: "Giving away" child psychology. *American Psychologist, 45*(12), 1325-1328.

The Role of Higher Education in Social Change, Public Policy and Community Collaboration

W. J. Blechman,
*Lawton & Rhea Chiles Center
for Healthy Mothers & Babies*

I have only been involved peripherally with higher education. As a physician in private practice, my contacts with universities were limited to taking courses to enhance my capabilities and teaching as part of the clinical faculty at the University of Miami Medical School as well as the Nova Southeastern School of Osteopathic Medicine. In my work for the State of Florida, I am a Courtesy Professor at the University of South Florida, but continue to have no role within the university itself. It is in part because of this lack of an internal relationship with universities that I was asked to present my views, as an "outsider," on the role that higher education is playing in social change, in public policy, and in community collaboration.

I recognize only indirect effects of higher education on social change. These effects are not as a result of direct institutional efforts and leadership. Instead, they result from one of the primary roles of a university, that is to prepare individuals to function appropriately in their chosen fields and in society. As for public policy, I am aware of some activity within academic institutions. However, I believe this involvement results from individual efforts, not as a result of institutional policy. On the other hand, I have been made aware of significant community collaborations. For example, my alma mater, Yale University, has been involved in a $50 million economic initiative with New Haven community interests. Further, other reports indicate that 180 institutions are involved in some type of partnerships, though I have no information on the quantity or quality of such efforts (*Wingspread Journal*, 1996).

I see a potential for higher education that I do not believe is being utilized. Instead of recognizing a corporate effort, I see only departmental or indeed individual activities in the areas of social change and public policy. I accept that community collaborations are occurring, but do not know the extent of these.

With regard to community collaboration, there is an increasing realization that programs or projects cannot simply be imposed upon communities and the people who live within. There is also an understanding that evaluation only of a community's needs (the deficit model) presents an overly restricted view of that neighborhood, town or other geographic structure. It is equally important to evaluate these entities for their assets and to learn how to make use of those assets to help create positive change. To accomplish this will require modifying the way we train those who will be responsible for evaluating conditions and initiating action. Thus, asset-based evaluations will need to be considered in university curricula, and further, practitioners will need to become increasingly capable of developing collaborative efforts.

Meanwhile, dramatic social changes have been and are continuing to occur. Welfare reform is only the most recent of these. An incomplete list might also include increases in divorce rate, numbers of single parent families, usage of illegal drugs and growing anti-government feelings. Whatever the examples picked, these changes require us to seriously examine our usual ways of affecting or modifying change. Meanwhile, public policy development in the United States appears too often to be driven by personal bias rather than by adequate research, and by money and the power of constituencies rather than by true need. The present investigations into the spending excesses and possible illegal acts by either or both major parties during the past presidential election suggest just how much special interests are willing to spend to influence policy, and how much they believe they can indeed do just that.

Perhaps part of the difficulty in assessing needs and creating social change and public policy arises as a result of contradictions that are a part of American society. We proclaim that we live in the land of the free, yet we have more persons in our jails per capita than any other nations with the possible exception of Russia. We quote Jefferson that "all men are created equal," ignoring the fact that children born to chemically addicted mothers living in poverty or those born with smaller brains due to malnutrition and those born to teenage mothers with poor parenting skills and even poorer resources cannot possibly be equal at their birth to most others. Nor will these children likely be exposed to a fraction of the opportunities available to others. We take pride in being able to provide the finest health care in the world, but will not acknowledge that lack of insurance prevents many of our citizens, including about 8.5 million children, from taking advantage of that care.

Perhaps our greatest contradiction, however, is we know some important preventable causes of illiteracy, school failure, crime, workplace failure, and welfare dependency, yet we show little willingness to put adequate resources into their prevention, or, at the very least, early intervention. Instead, we will spend money attempting expensive and often only partially effective late interventions. I include neo-natal intensive care units as well as prisons in this latter category. Perhaps a year or two ago I watched a television show that had to do with the prison systems in this country. Towards the end of the show there was an interview with the executive director of the Texas Department of Corrections who was asked if there weren't some things that could be done to keep more people out of prison. His first comment was that perhaps we as a nation were being penny-wise and pound-foolish. "We probably should be putting more money into Head Start," he said.

In my opinion, centers of higher education can and should add significantly more to the discourse that leads to public policy development and social change in addition to actively collaborating with communities. To do this, however, requires that each institution evaluate its resources to determine in what areas it might become involved most effectively.

Let me use an area of personal interest as an example of how centers of higher education might be more effective in the public policy/social change areas. For several years I have been involved in issues related to early childhood and consider it important to develop a major societal focus on children, aged 0-3, and their families, and efforts to prevent problems in these groups. The idea is not new. Human development researchers, pediatricians, police chiefs, juvenile court judges, corrections officials, and increasing numbers of educators have recognized the poor outcomes resulting from a general lack of understanding about the importance of this period of human life, yet there has been remarkably little translation into effective public policy.

The past several years have been providing a steady flow of remarkable findings about the developing human brain, findings that have profound implications. Once considered to be an impenetrable black box, the living brain gradually is yielding its secrets to technological advances. Neuroscientists are confirming the interplay of genes and environment in directing a brain's development. They are showing how undeveloped the human brain is at birth and that it is within the first three years that the brain stores information and memories that create the foundation for later learning.

According to Kotulak (1996), "Two of the most surprising and profound discoveries [by researchers] are that the brain uses the outside world to shape itself and that it goes through crucial periods in which brain cells must have appropriate stimulation to develop such powers as vision, language, smell, muscle control, and reasoning" (p. 3). Equally powerful is the confirmation of nurturing as the basis for developing the brain's centers for emotion and the need to enhance not only cognitive intelligence, but emotional intelligence as well. This information points strongly to the importance of early attachment, the parent's mental health, and the quality of care (or lack of quality) given by caregivers. Our colleagues are showing us that neglect as well as chronic stress can actually change the structure of the developing brain. Increasingly, scientists are able to identify certain dysfunctional areas within the brain, for example in auditory processing, which offers an understanding of the pathogenesis leading to certain functional deficits, some of which may be reversible.

Language skills are acquired earlier than previously recognized. The importance of enhancing the development of these skills and the long-term negative effects resulting from lack of appropriate stimulation for such development—whether by disease, family dysfunction, congenital abnormalities, or neglect—are being increasingly recognized. Studies confirm that lack of stimulation of the brain may lead to a smaller organ, one that may be associated with developmental delays of varying severity.

What can centers of higher education do with this information to help communities and the nation? In a center with a strong applied developmental science focus in the area of early childhood, I can foresee a deliberate effort by the administration of the university to bring together individuals from other departments in a joint effort to utilize the research results and skills of the former along with the disciplines of the latter. In the case of early childhood, I can visualize expanded value by adding research and/or practical considerations from departments involving ethics, economics, communications, management, education, public health, management information systems, marketing and perhaps others.

This would be in addition to the role of the center in supporting its faculty and stimulating departmental research and teaching. While these are obviously obligatory, they are an incomplete response on the part of the organization and potentially waste an opportunity. While faculty perform research in areas where they have specialized interest and teach students in their area of expertise, these same faculty cannot be expert in other subject matter areas. By combining the knowledge and experience of various disciplines, I believe it may be possible for those in higher education to have a greater impact on social change and public policy.

At the same time, a university could bring together those with skills which would enhance integrative program development, working with government, business, and local organizations. In some instances, it may be necessary to look outside the university for the most qualified person or persons for this particular expertise. These various skills can also be used to identify and subsequently reduce duplication of effort within the community. Additionally, this could stimulate a much more rapid passage of information to that subset of individuals or groups for whom this information should be especially meaningful as well as to the general public.

While not all might share my particular interest in issues related to young children and the steadily increasing understanding of brain development in this area, I doubt that anyone would deny the importance of recent neuroscientific findings. These findings are particularly challenging in view of the recent changes in this nation's welfare system. There is general agreement that getting and keeping women off of welfare requires the availability of child care. However, recent studies of family child care (the type most frequently used for infants and toddlers) in three communities found 56% of the homes to be adequate/custodial, while 35% were rated as inadequate (growth harming). Only 9% were considered to be growth enhancing (Galinsky, Howes, Kontos & Shinn, 1994). Further, a report by the Committee for Economic Development (1993), refers to a study of center-based child care, noting that quality was barely adequate. While one cannot generalize to the rest of the country, indications are that large numbers of children lack quality, defined by appropriate stimulation and responsiveness, as well as safety in their child care settings.

I believe that centers of higher education should involve themselves actively in the training of child care workers, with an emphasis on child development and brain development, especially during the first few years of life. Students should be encouraged to spend time in child care settings. Offers should be made to enhance knowledge of the recent research in brain development within school and preschool educators, and also school board members. Furthermore, the university or college should approach organizations, such as Zero to Three, the Families and Work Institute, among others, which are involved in advocacy to determine possible common interests and directions. While interested faculty or administrators presently link with such organizations, I believe that a more formal approach from the institution itself offers the greatest opportunity for involvement that will lead to significant policy and social change.

I assume that my recommendations would require changes in the ways that centers of higher education presently operate. It might also add to the workload of faculty members and administration. However, I believe universities and colleges have an obligation to the communities in which they exist, and that they should make the greatest use of their faculty and other staff. In my particular point of interest, there is also an obligation which may well affect each of us through our children and grandchildren.

REFERENCES

Committee for Economic Development. (1993). Why child care matters: Preparing young children for a more productive America. A statement by the Research and Policy Committee of the Committee for Economic Development. New York: Committee for Economic Development.

Galinsky, E., Howes, C., Kontos, S. & Shinn, M. (1994). *The study of children in family child care and relative care*. New York: Families and Work Institute.

Kotulak, R. (1996). *Inside the brain*. Kansas City, MO: Andrews and McMeel.

Wingspread Journal. (1996). Communities and universities join to revitalize cities? *Wingspread Journal, 18*(4), 11-13.

Fostering Linkages with the University in Public Policy Engagement

Jack Levine, *Center for Florida's Children*
Barbara Ash, *Florida State University*

THE CASE FOR COLLABORATION

If ever the time was right to build bridges between human development scholars and the discipline's practitioners in the community in which the university sits, it is now. Despite advances made by scholars and practitioners in early childhood development, child maltreatment and neglect intervention, access to preventive health care, and teen-pregnancy prevention, these complex issues continue to challenge our communities. Sadly, proactive collaboration between practitioners and scholars in their search for solutions is rare. That must change if we are to influence public policy and attract funding that will help us find viable remedies to these social ills.

Confronted with mounting challenges from government and policy makers to prove our relevance and demonstrate results, we are vulnerable to knife-wielding lawmakers intent on cutting programs or research projects that fail to produce dividends on their investment. In addition, now more than ever before, private philanthropists, deluged with requests, are scrutinizing grant proposals with an eye for cost-benefit and accountability measures that show the positive impact of the financial investment in services.

Certainly, professions that look for root causes and emphasize prevention and early intervention are in a most precarious position: statistics rarely tell us how many children did *not* die from maltreatment because of parental training programs, or how many babies were *not* born prematurely because their mothers had pre-natal care, or how many adolescents did *not* commit a crime because an after-school program kept them off the streets. Diplomat Henry Kissinger once said, "The history of things that *didn't* happen never gets written."

Especially in a climate of fiscal conservatism, investors want to immediately see what their money has bought. Explaining that a five, ten, or even 20-year time frame for evidence of effectiveness to emerge may result in blank stares from officials who think in much shorter time-frames. Like one pundit quipped, "Don't ask elected officials to impact the next generation if their sole focus is on the next election."

Human development scholars and practitioners know there have been dividends from society's investment in children and families: reduced costs in medical care, more successful schooling, fewer consequences of crime, and economic deficits from lost income. But these results are rarely immediate. Savvy investors know, however, that the true value on investment is in long-term gain. The same applies to investment in the health, stability and security of children and families.

Such a message is a hard sell to decision-makers who tend to allocate resources to fixing, rather than to preventing problems, but it is a message that we must communicate clearly and consistently.

The audiences we must influence are powerful:

Community, state and national leaders who make statutory, budgetary and program decisions that affect children and families;

Media professionals who decide what is "news," what gets front-page play or prime-time coverage, and what is ignored; and

The 30 percent of eligible voters who cast ballots, and therefore, are most influential with elected officials (see group one, above).

We can never assume that everyone in our target audiences is willing to discuss certain social issues. Some policy makers are super-sensitive about confronting issues like alcohol or drug addiction or domestic violence because those are human behaviors that transcend economic and racial lines. In very many cases, these are not just "someone else's problem," but may well hit too close to home for comfort. Let us remember that denial of a problem is the fastest way to ignore responsibility for action. That's true both personally and politically.

Influencing public policy and program development in the human behavior arena is a tremendous challenge because many of the issues surrounding family dysfunction have traditionally been more the realm of "private" than "public" concern. It's nearly impossible to reach consensus on a solution if there is scant acknowledgment that a problem exists, can be statistically documented, and can gain the interest of a sufficiently powerful constituency to call for action.

For example, spouse abuse and child maltreatment have been social problems for centuries, but only recently have become public policy issues. Why this transformation from the intensely private to an openly public outcry for action? First, media reporting of especially egregious cases of maltreatment have caught the attention of newspaper readers and television news viewers. The shock value of learning about the brutal treatment of defenseless infants, or the repeated beatings by a spouse who has broken the vow to "love and cherish," motivates outrage and creates a demand for response.

The challenge, however, is hubbed in the fact that social and behavioral issues are more complex than the usual "crime and punishment" methodology of law and policy. These are sensitive issues which require more than the reflex reaction of putting the perpetrator behind bars. While there are certain domestic crimes that demand criminal prosecution, the broad range of negative social behaviors have, at their point of origin, a life-long exposure to maltreatment, emotional turmoil, and factors such as drug and alcohol addiction, mental disturbance, or severe mental incapacity. While these mitigating factors do not excuse the resultant behavior, they go a long way toward explaining it. And the opportunities for prevention, intervention, and perhaps treatment, through creative public policy initiatives, would serve the community better in the long run that sole reliance on criminal justice processing and incarceration. By analogy, "If your only tool is a hammer, everything looks like a nail." So, too, by presenting multiple policy options, rooted in the social and behavioral sciences, a more enlightened and successful set of solutions in both law and budget will be found.

To achieve effective human development policy goals, we must recognize that access to science-based information is critical. We cannot just *say* something works. We have to prove that a policy initiative, a program model, or a set of strategic actions in the community works to achieve a documented outcome. This is the critical role that scientific social research plays. Research serves not only as a source of valid "cause and effect" relationships, but also provides the analysis of intervening factors that influence human behavior and family interaction. Used this way, research provides the leverage to influence policymakers. One can imagine a lever wedged against a wheel that provides the pressure to lift the wheel. Viewed similarly, well-founded research applies pressure, or compelling evidence, that enables policymakers to make informed decisions.

It is prudent to understand that policy makers like to make decisions—"that's their job." We should never appear to be poised to make decisions for them. What we can do, however, is to present policy makers with options which are solidly supported by scientific evidence and stated clearly so that the decisions they make have a prospect of success. If that method is employed, progress will be reached.

Responsible policy makers who understand the importance of addressing the identified problem, and respect the reliability of the information they are provided, may well see it in their interest to respond positively to create solutions.

COLLABORATION: A TEAM SPORT

Effective advocacy is a team sport in which the diversity of each member's strengths, style and substance, and how well each covers his or her position, is key. Obviously, the team play needs to be coordinated. The Human Development Team is comprised of three groups:

> Practitioners—committed individuals who work on the frontline to meet the economic, social and psychological needs of children and families. This group includes social workers, early childhood development specialists, psychologists, child care workers, family and consumer sciences professionals and health care professionals.

> Organizations—committed to civic service and policy change, some of which are very community-based, such as neighborhood associations, while others have national affiliations, such as the Urban League. Some (e.g., the Center for Florida's Children) are advocacy specialists who have a network of colleagues all over the nation and work cooperatively with the diverse Florida advocate community. Their stock and trade is leveraging the expertise and the experience of individuals, through strategic media communications and grassroots outreach, to affect policy change.

> Human Development Scholars—experts who possess valuable knowledge based on authoritative research. Of all the academic disciplines, human development is most conducive to advocacy, community action, and policy change. Academic leaders in this field have available to them in the community for study newborns, toddlers, teenagers, elders and families who are oftentimes ready, willing and able, as recipients of services, to assist in positive research activities.

Human development scholars and practitioners can learn strategies and skills from each other, but it takes practice. It is in our best interest—and certainly in the interest of children and families—to take advantage of the wealth of knowledge each possesses. Scholars do not have to be comfortable giving *barn burner* speeches, or testifying at the Capitol to contribute positively to public outreach and policy initiatives. Those who are at ease giving community speeches need the substantive base provided by the scientific findings in which their message is firmly rooted.

As teammates, we possess knowledge and insight that can guide powerful people to make correct decisions. In fact, it is our duty to provide policy makers with the research-based knowledge and firsthand experience critical in shaping policies and programs that can address the root of family and children's concerns.

Few public officials are experts on all the issues about which they will make decisions. We should never assume that their personal staffs, who focus most of their energy on constituent problems, can help them make totally informed policy decisions. Unless we take the initiative, public officials' decisions will continue to be heavily influenced by their political advisors, the people with whom they socialize, or the people who gave campaign contributions. Those individuals rarely are experts in the human services field.

When those closest to public officials have as limited experience on the issues as the official has, the quality of the work product usually suffers. Bad public policy is usually the result of a handful of horrible anecdotes, misinterpreted by people who know little about the circumstances, and acted upon by people who are looking for the easy answer to complex problems. When it comes time to write laws, amend statutes, or pass budgets that affect social policy, we should never assume that our public officials know all they need to know to make informed choices. Experts, by virtue of their scientific research knowledge, or practitioners who have a solid base of experience, must be willing to fill the void if progress is to be achieved.

Similar perspectives are true with relationships in the journalism community. It is a reporter or editor's job to cultivate reliable sources who can give access to information and help interpret the mass of data into a digestible 10-20-inch newspaper story, or a 30-second broadcast soundbite. While many in the field of human development assume that media professionals have a Rolodex brimming with sources, the reality is that responsible journalists are always in the hunt for fresh ideas, new information, and exciting angles on the news of the day. It is incumbent upon research scholars, community practitioners, and advocates, to develop proactive relationships with print and broadcast media professionals so that the reporting of news and the crafting of opinion is as factual and inspirational as possible.

By honing the skills of strategic communications, scholars and practitioners can achieve two important goals: 1) getting the word out about the importance of their work to a broad audience of potential supporters, and 2) influencing the very policy makers who govern us. Political leaders are gluttonous consumers of the news; they intensely need to know if someone is complimenting them, or complaining about them, in the morning paper or on the evening news. When human development professionals, volunteers, and the families served are in the news, and good information about their achievements are public knowledge, then positive public policy attention will be the predictable outcome.

While there are numerous organizations and individuals in the community with whom social science faculty can collaborate, a key group must never be left out of the public policy equation: human development students sitting in seats in their classroom. Properly informed and inspired, human development students can become a powerful population of advocates who are energetic and eager to practice what they are learning to affect positive community change. Certainly, they need to develop the right tools, but they have the main ingredient: enthusiasm.

Faculty can build a foundation for advocacy by gearing the curriculum, project assignments and internships to develop the basic and advanced skills of advocacy. There is no more powerful introduction to the need for change than giving students the opportunity to work in the community on behalf of senior citizens or children, or a social program serving families or teens at risk. While many of these programs are places of enormous energy and achievement, there is the reality that most community-based health, human service and family programs operate with minimal resources and are constantly under pressure to recruit and retain qualified staff, and to provide a high level of care under stressful circumstances.

With this direct service experience as a guide, the skills of communication, problem analysis, solution development, and agenda building for change can be the positive, practical activity of students who aspire to become human service professionals. Community voices, both from the volunteer and professional organization perspective, should be frequent visitors to human development classrooms, giving their "real world" perspectives on policy and program, and guiding students to see the ways they can be powerful agents for both case and class advocacy.

In collaboration with other disciplines within the university community, human development professionals can create exciting projects for replication in other locales and university settings. For example, just one block from the College of Human Sciences on the campus of Florida State University stands one of the highest-rated film and broadcast schools in the nation. These two disciplines could be working together to show on film the importance of arms that hug, the miracle of legs that run, the joy a healthy baby can bring, and the success that can come from a good education.

Collaborations across the disciplines—education and law; medicine and communications; human development and political science—can enrich the experience of students, invigorate the creativity of faculty, and produce a high level of policy and program initiatives which would improve the quality of life for the community.

CONCLUSION

With the government, taxpayers and philanthropists demanding more accountability for their investment in research and social programs, scholars and practitioners in the field of human development are under pressure to prove their positive impact on society.

It is in the best interest of both the scholarly and practitioner communities to develop the strategies and skills necessary to build successful partnerships, broaden the audiences with whom they communicate, and empower students and community contacts to take a more active role in affecting policies and programs that can benefit children and families.

Public Policy: Roles for Faculty
Clara Pratt, *Oregon State University*

To implement effective public policy education, faculty in human sciences must understand their unique resources and potential roles. These faculty roles parallel the dimensions of academic scholarship defined by Boyer (1990) in *Scholarship Reconsidered*:

> . . . scholarship means engaging in original research. But the work of scholarship also means stepping back from one's investigation, looking for connections, building bridges between theory and practice, and communicating one's knowledge effectively . . . (p. 16)

This chapter builds upon Boyer's notion of scholarship to highlight four faculty roles in policy—the scholarship of discovery, the scholarship of integration, the scholarship of application, and the scholarship of teaching.

Although each form of scholarship is detailed separately, it is important to remember that they are *fundamentally related*. For example, the scholarship of discovery or research is based in part on the scholarship of integration which considers results across earlier studies to establish underlying patterns and to define unanswered questions. Similarly the scholarship of teaching is enriched by the other forms of scholarship.

The specific focus of this chapter is on forms of scholarship applied to family policy, that is, how government policies affect families (Aldous & Dumon, 1991; Zimmerman, 1992a). Family policy addresses the issues that affect individuals and families over the lifespan. These issues include poverty and economic vulnerability, parenting and parent education and support, child and dependent care, teen pregnancy and parenting, grandparenting and grandparents' rights, domestic violence, family preservation and child protection, and a wide range of other concerns. It is in the arena of family policy that most human sciences faculty and professionals will find greatest relevance.

To effectively advocate for policies that will support individuals and families requires a clear vision of families and individuals across the lifespan. This vision must present strengths as well as challenges, recognize diversity, and illuminate the impact of socioeconomic contexts on well-being (Fine, 1992; Rodman & Sidden, 1992; Wisensale, 1992; Zimmerman, 1992b). This vision must also build upon empirical knowledge (Pratt, 1995). For example, in their excellent review of the consequences of poverty for children, Duncan and Brooks-Gunn (1997) move beyond rhetoric to research findings in order to illuminate how poverty affects development especially in the early years. They conclude with a discussion of how policies, affecting income transfer programs, health care, and early childhood care and education, can improve the life chances of children who live in poor families. This review creates a clear vision of how poverty impacts children and exemplifies the union of the scholarship of discovery, integration, and application.

SCHOLARSHIP OF DISCOVERY

The scholarship of discovery is one of the most valuable roles that faculty play in reference to policy. A strong research base distinguishes applied human developmental science from other voices in the policy arena. This research base enables human sciences faculty to be exceptionally well prepared to inform policy questions. For example, the policy debate about teen pregnancy is often waged over values. In contrast, human sciences faculty can bring empirically-based information to discussions of the dynamics of teen pregnancy and the effectiveness of various approaches to the reduction of teen pregnancy (Chase-Lansdale & Brooks-Gunn, 1996; Jorgensen, Potts & Camp, 1993; Zabin & Hayward, 1993). Faculty contribute to the empirical base of knowledge about human development policy options through applied research, policy analysis, and program evaluation.

Applied research. By generating knowledge that has clear implications for action and policy, applied research builds the capability to address human problems. Applied research must be based on conceptual perspectives that go beyond "satisfy(ing) our intellectual curiosity . . . to instigate effective social policy, improve the quality of marriages and family life, and help emancipate those who are locked into unfair or oppressive structures" (Sprey, 1991, p. 130).

Because no one discipline can be sensitive to all potentially relevant variables, policy research demands an interdisciplinary approach which is the hallmark of applied developmental science (Lerner & Fisher, 1994). Applied developmental science provides a particularly valuable interdisciplinary framework for policy research because it builds on three critical perspectives: life-span development, human ecology, and developmental contextualism (Lerner & Fisher, 1994). First, the life-span perspective conceptualizes development as occurring throughout life, in parents as well as children and in the elderly as well as the young. Earlier development influences later development and contributes greatly to diversity and individual differences. For policy, the life-span perspective establishes the importance of individual differences and the relevance of prevention, early intervention, and remediation strategies throughout the life cycle. Human ecology and developmental contextualism embed the development and behavior of individuals and family units within social, cultural, economic, and physical environments. These perspectives are particularly relevant to policy because development and well-being are conceptualized as the result of dynamic, reciprocal interactions between individuals and their environments. Many of these environments are directly influenced by education, employment, welfare, health care, housing, justice, and other public policies.

To be most relevant to policy and program development, applied research must investigate variables that are amenable to change or that mediate change. While demographic, individual, and intra-family level variables are important to describe and understand a social problem, alone they are insufficient to guide policy and program development. The social environments created by culture, communities, service systems, and economics must also be addressed. Using an applied developmental science approach, scholars can effectively conceptualize research in terms of individual and environmental or contextual variables that are amenable to change.

For example, research that addresses both individual and contextual level variables is most likely to influence policies and programs that reduce welfare dependence (Cubbins, 1992; Ellwood, 1988; Funiciello, 1993; Webster, Hu & Weeks, 1993). Such conceptualizations of welfare reform will include individual level variables (e.g., education, work skills, and work experience) and critical contextual variables (e.g., the availability of child and health care, child support enforcement, local employment rates, and wage and benefit levels). Similarly, research on the effects of poverty on children (Duncan & Brooks-Gunn, 1997; Brooks-Gunn, Duncan & Aber, 1997) has clarified the individual, family, educational, and neighborhood variables that are associated with positive and negative outcomes for children. From this work, policy implications can be clearly drawn.

Policy analysis. Public policies provide the conceptual frameworks for government's approach to social problems. These frameworks reflect policy makers' beliefs about particular social problems, as well as societal values, and perceived alternative policy options (Zimmerman, 1992a). Policy analysis aims to discover and define the relationships among social needs and social, economic, bureaucratic, and political possibilities and actions (Unrau, 1994).

Analysis of family policies is an important pursuit in the scholarship of discovery (Aldous & Dumon, 1991; Monroe, 1987). Policy analysis is also valuable to the scholarship of integration and the scholarship of application. As a research activity, however, the focus of policy analysis is the *understanding* of particular public policies, rather than on action to change or influence policies. Policy analysis often includes historical research that traces the history and dynamics of various policies. For example, historical policy analysis is a central tool in recent investigations of family life (Coontz, 1992; Zimmerman, 1992a), family economic status (Mishel & Bernstein, 1993) and welfare in the United States (Funiciello, 1993; Bane & Ellwood, 1994.)

Program evaluation. Programs are the specific interventions that operationalize a policy. Program evaluation is focused on determining the operation and impact of a specific intervention (Unrau, 1994). Program evaluation can provide invaluable information about one incarnation of a policy. Evaluation must include an excellent description of the program's objectives, activities, intended clients, success in reaching the intended clients, and outcomes for various clients. Together, policy analysis and program evaluation offer a comprehensive assessment of the context, operation, and outcomes of a policy and its related programs (Unrau, 1994).

In summary, faculty can make powerful contributions to policy through applied research, policy analysis, and program evaluation. Findings from such scholarly work can be used to inform programs and policies. Because faculty are often seen as experts, they can have great credibility with policy makers (Aldous & Dumon, 1991). This is especially true when faculty scholarship addresses important social issues and is effectively communicated. Such communication links the scholarship of discovery with the scholarship of integration and scholarship of application. It is to these forms of scholarship that we turn next.

SCHOLARSHIP OF INTEGRATION

Looking for connections between theory, research, and practice is the essential task of the scholarship of integration (Boyer, 1990). As noted earlier, the scholarship of integration, which synthesizes results across various perspectives and studies, is essential to all other forms of scholarship—discovery, application, and teaching. For example, every effective study begins with a review of earlier work in order to define approaches, identify patterns, and clarify unanswered questions. Similarly, program evaluations typically begin with a comprehensive review of related research and evaluation studies. Thus the scholarship of integration is essential to the scholarship of discovery.

The scholarship of integration is also critical to effectively inform public policy. Recent comprehensive reviews of research have addressed several contemporary policy issues, including adolescent drug and alcohol use (Hawkins, Catalano & Miller, 1992), adolescent sexual behavior (Chase-Lansdale & Brooks-Gunn, 1994;

Hardy & Zabin, 1991; Miller & Moore, 1991), family health and health care (Price & Elliott, 1993), family caregiving in chronic illness (Biegel, Sales & Schulz, 1991), and other social needs (see, for example, Lerner & Fisher, 1994; Olson & Hanson, 1990). Very importantly, these interdisciplinary reviews integrate results *across* various studies to define underlying patterns and fundamental perspectives.

Similarly, comprehensive integration of conclusions *across* program evaluations are needed to inform decision making about programs and policies. Such integrative reviews have been published on several issues including early family support and delinquency (Yoshikawa, 1994), family violence (Gelles & Conte, 1991), family caregiving (Biegel, Sales & Schulz, 1991), adolescent drug use (Pentz, 1996), adolescent pregnancy and teen parenthood (Chase-Lansdale & Brooks-Gunn, 1996; Zabin & Hayward, 1993), and other interventions. Continued scholarly integration across evaluations is vital to guide future program and policy development.

In addition, products from the scholarship of integration may be published and disseminated by advocacy organizations, state agencies, and universities themselves. These outlets may provide faster "turn-around" than formal academic presses; speed is often critical to relevance and use in policy decision-making. Recent examples of such publications are *Building Results: From Wellness Goods to Measurable Outcomes for Oregon's Children* (Pratt, Katzev, Henderson & Ozretich, 1997) published by the Oregon Commission on Children and Families to guide statewide performance planning and measurement. Another example is the *Utah Sourcebook on Aging* (Wright, 1998). Published by the University of Utah Gerontology Center, this sourcebook is an overview of demographic and policy issues in Utah and the intermountain West.

Finally, in the past two decades, the scholarship of integration has advanced from primarily qualitative analyses to include quantitative meta-analytic procedures. Meta-analysis statistically analyzes results from a set of quantitative studies in order to compare outcomes across samples, measurement approaches, and other methodological variations (see Cooper & Hedges, 1994). Recent published meta-analyses have focused upon teen pregnancy prevention (Franklin, Grant, Corcoran, Miller & Bultman, 1997), juvenile delinquency (Lipsey, 1992; Lipsey & Wilson, 1993), community psychology (Durlak & Lipsey, 1991), family therapy (Shadish, 1992), and other areas. Today the scholarship of integration can effectively use both qualitative, conceptual analysis *and* quantitative, meta-analytic techniques.

SCHOLARSHIP OF APPLICATION

Building bridges between theory, research, and practice is the essential task of the scholarship of application (Boyer, 1990). The scholarship of application seeks to influence the policies, programs, and other environments that affect children, youth, and families. To influence policy, faculty must inform the political process that is *essential* in policy decision-making. Through the political process, strategies for addressing human problems are formulated and agreed upon out of a massive complexity of values, problems, possible solutions, and resources (Lindbloom & Woodhouse, 1993). Without a political process, "sheer information and reasoning alone would have to be sufficient to bring all the relevant parties together" (Lindbloom & Woodhouse, 1993, p. 16). Faculty can participate in the political process through the scholarship of application, including such activities as public policy education, advocacy, and advisory service.

Preceding public policy education, advocacy, and advisory service, careful analysis of policies and statutes is essential (Monroe, 1987; Coyne, 1993). In the scholarship of application, policy and statutory analyses are used to assess policy proposals in order to inform the public and other decision-makers about the likely impact on families of proposed policies and statutes. Focused on application, policy and statutory analysis asks questions such as: Is this proposed policy or statute empirically valid in terms of its causal model? What other variables (e.g., cultural, social, economic, or technological) will affect the outcome and the implementation of the statute? Policy and statutory analyses may also include the application of family policy criteria. Family policy criteria are based on beliefs about what would be the desirable impact of policies upon families (Stevens, 1992). One set of family criteria established by the U.S. House Select Sub-Committee on Children, Youth, and Families maintains that family policies and programs should:

1. Encourage and reinforce family, parental, and marital stability, especially when children are involved.
2. Support and supplement, rather than substitute for, family functioning.
3. Recognize the strength and persistence of family ties, even when they are problematic.
4. Treat families as partners when providing services to individuals and strengthen families' capacity to fulfill their social roles and tasks.
5. Recognize the diversity of family life.
6. Recognize that families in the greatest social and economic need and those most vulnerable to breakdown should be the primary priority for government policies and programs. (Stevens, 1992; U.S. House Select Sub-Committee, 1986)

These principles have implications for the many current issues in family policy. For example, family preservation policies (Cole & Duva, 1990) certainly reflect the first three of these principles. The fourth principle (treating families as partners when providing services to individuals) is central to the family support movement (Kagan & Weissbourd, 1994) and to programs such as dependent care, respite, and in home services. Similar principles have been articulated by other governmental (Goetz & Peck, 1994) and advocacy organizations (Weissbourd, 1994). For example, the Premier's Council in Support of Alberta (Canada) Families (1993) has formulated several principles into a "family policy grid," to provide a framework for assessing the potential impact of *all* provincial government policies on families.

Clearly, in the process of selecting criteria, some principles are included while others are omitted. For example, in the family criteria listed above (U.S. House Select Sub-Committee, 1986), the principle of family stability is included while individual rights is not. However, the principle of family stability does not argue that, in all circumstances, family stability is desirable. Rather, the principle asks scholars and policy makers to consider: What will be this policy's likely impact on family stability? Family criteria assure that the possible impacts of policies and programs on families are considered.

Public policy education. Once scholars have a clear vision of policy issues, policies and statutes, an important activity in the scholarship of application is public policy education. Public policy education provides citizens and decision-makers with information about the political process as well as the content of specific policy issues and options (Boyle & Mulcahy, 1993). Such education is essential. Many citizens have little understanding of how to effectively participate in the political process. Education about the political process and how to effectively participate in this process is now common at professional meeting such as the National Council of Family Relations, as well as through Extension and other education programs (Stevens, 1992).

In addition, most citizens, and many legislators and elected officials, have little understanding of specific policy issues and options for addressing these issues

(Boyle & Mulcahy, 1993; Lindbloom & Woodhouse, 1993). Thus education is needed that provides neutral, accurate information about specific policy issues. This education enables decision-makers to make more informed political choices. For such public policy education to be valued, position papers, fact sheets, letters to the editor, and community forums must utilize a factual, informative approach. For example, the Oregon State University Extension Service developed a fact sheet and community forum series on a highly controversial death with dignity initiative measure facing Oregon voters in November, 1994 (Hare, et al., 1994). The group of faculty and professionals who jointly developed the fact sheet and program held very different opinions on the issue and worked to achieve a factual, informative approach. Such policy education is essential to building political knowledge among the citizens and other decision-makers.

Family Impact Seminars offer a forum for policy education that is designed especially for policy makers. The goal of Family Impact Seminars is to provide objective, non-partisan information on family issues. This information synthesizes research on the topic and summarizes a range of policy options in light of this research. Typically the seminars include short forums supported by an extensively researched briefing report (see for example, Ooms & Weintaub, 1992; Ooms, Cohen & Hutchins, 1995). Originally developed to address federal policy, the seminar format has been effectively adapted to support state legislators and other state and local officials in several states. For example, Wisconsin's Family Impact Seminars have attracted over 100 participants and have addressed issues such as single parenthood and children's well-being, juvenile crime prevention, welfare reform, child support, and teen pregnancy prevention (Bogenschneider, 1995). Such federal, state, and local seminars for policy makers offer important forums for applying knowledge in policy arena.

Advocacy. In addition to public policy education, faculty can exercise the scholarship of application through advocacy efforts. Appropriate advocacy activities are legally defined for employees of government and most non-profit agencies (Trister & Weill, 1991). Because many faculty are publicly employed, knowledge of the general nature of these laws and rules is essential. In most states, laws prohibit public employees from advocacy that involves direct lobbying or using public resources to influence an election or the adoption of a particular piece of legislation. Generally, these laws note that these restrictions should *not* limit the full exercise of citizenship in a personal capacity.

Under the federal law several advocacy activities are *not* considered lobbying (Trister & Weill, 1991). Among these advocacy activities are public policy education or reports that provide sufficient information for persons to draw their own conclusions, technical advice or assistance that is requested by legislative bodies, communication about how legislation would affect one's own organization, and commenting on agency regulations or rules. Finally, advocacy on broad social issues, rather than specific legislation, is not defined as lobbying. It is in this arena that faculty can advocate for recognition and support of children, youth, and family issues.

Advisory and participatory roles. Faculty can make very important policy contributions through service on governmental and private sector advisory groups. These range from local nursing home boards to state level commissions on families to national corporations or foundations. Commissions and other advisory groups are created for many purposes and range from visible but weak political appointment, to groups with significant influence over legislative agendas and agency actions. All states and localities have important policy advisory groups that address the concerns of human development. Some groups carry a broad charge such as keeping the issues of children, families, or the elderly in the minds of the public (and policy makers) and working to create political support for policies and programs. Other groups have a narrower, specific focus, such as homelessness, domestic violence, teen pregnancy prevention, or child-care.

Because of this range of purposes and strengths, faculty must carefully review opportunities for advisory service and consider the mission, membership, and power of the group, as well as the time commitment required. Faculty who are new to advisory groups may find that participation on local boards or on shorter-term ad hoc technical committees offers excellent opportunities to explore the nature and dynamics of advisory efforts.

Finally, faculty can participate in local, state, national, and even international policy conferences. Policy conferences offer forums in which faculty can interact with and influence policy makers and advocates. At some policy conferences, faculty will find opportunities to present and apply research findings, much like the Family Impact Seminars. In addition, participation in policy conferences assures that faculty are exposed to the "front-line" concerns and issues facing policy makers and program administrators. This exposure can enrich the scholarship of discovery and of teaching.

Many professional organizations, such as the National Council on Family Relations and the American Society on Aging offer conference tracks that focus on policy issues. Other opportunities for participation are found at local and state summit meetings, governor's conferences, legislative forums, advocacy forums, among others. National meetings such as the White House Conference on Aging offer significant opportunities for faculty who have demonstrated substantial interest and commitment to advocacy and political participation. International meetings, such as the United Nation's sponsored NGO (non-governmental organization) forums, typically involve both official delegates who represent their countries governments and other participants who represent a wide range of NGO institutions and groups. For example, at the UN 4th Conference on Women held in Beijing, China in 1996, participants included 1,500 official national delegates and over 30,000 others, including faculty from colleges and universities around the world.

Communication in the scholarship of application. Faculty can contribute to policy only if their perspectives are effectively communicated to policy makers (Haskins, 1993). The under-utilization of research and evaluation information in policymaking has been recognized for two decades (Rich, 1979). If policies are to be influenced by research and evaluation findings, faculty must be professionally and personally committed to communicating with decision-makers, legislative aides and other staff, and advocates (Shadish, Cook & Leviton, 1991). Effective communication with policy makers demands that faculty recognize that it is *their* responsibility to communicate in a way that policy makers can understand and utilize (Aldous & Dumon, 1991). Sending reprints will not suffice!

Policy makers act on more issues in a single year than any one person could begin to understand. In the U.S. House of Representatives nearly 10,000 domestic policy bills are discussed annually ranging from water quality and environmental protection to welfare reform and education (Lindbloom & Woodhouse, 1993). In 1997, state legislatures addressed hundreds of bills affecting children, youth, and families across the lifespan. For example, a review of child-related bills introduced in state legislatures in 1997 included such topics as Aid to Families with Dependent Children (AFDC), Temporary Assistance to Needy Families (TANF), children's protective services, family preservation, teen pregnancy and parenting, juvenile justice, health care and health care financing, and early childhood education and child care (National Conference on State Legislatures, 1998).

In order to respond to this massive workload, federal and state legislative policy makers often specialize in particular issues and rely on a complex system of committees, sub-committees, and staffs to review, refine, and filter legislation.

Understanding the system by which issues become proposed legislation and then law is critical to effective communication with policy makers. Monroe (1991) provided family professionals with a solid primer on this complicated process, pointing out the opportunities for input, including during interim periods when legislators are not in formal session.

Information overload is a debilitating problem for policy makers. For communications to be powerful and influential, faculty must recognize this reality. While the academic world emphasizes inquiry, detail, data, and first authorship, the policy world emphases action, feasibility, simplification, intuition, and coalitions (Pratt, 1995). Given these differing views, effective communication requires faculty's careful thought and commitment. Simplification of ideas, reports, briefings, and recommendations is essential (Gove & Knott, 1994; Haskins, 1993; Ooms, 1993). Detailed backup support should be available, but the essence of each communication must be clear and concise.

Effective language includes clear descriptions and definitions, avoids jargon, translates complex ideas and statistics into common language and examples, and summarizes major concepts. Implications and recommendations should be clearly related to data but highlighted in a separate area of the report or briefing. In sum, academics, who are accustomed to explaining every word and presenting detailed statistical analyses, will find that effective communication demands a new approach that emphasizes accurate summaries, descriptions that paint powerful pictures, and clearly stated implications (Pratt, 1995).

SCHOLARSHIP OF TEACHING

What should faculty teach students about policy? All of the *processes* presented earlier in this chapter, including applied research, advocacy roles, the legislative process, and communication techniques, are potentially important topics for students. In addition, many faculty can profitably address *content* of policy issues, such as economic vulnerability and welfare reform, family law, teen pregnancy and parenting, early childhood care and education, health and well-being across the lifespan, and other topics. Building from an applied developmental science perspective, courses will investigate the individual and environmental contexts of these issues. Several earlier chapters detail guidelines for undergraduate and graduate curriculum including experiential learning and other instructional approaches (see chapters by Ley, Craig, McClintock & Wilcox). In addition, policy curriculum and instructional resources have been well-described by Fisher (1993), Anderson and Skinner (1995), and Skinner and Anderson (1993).

Across these fine works, one theme is clear: The scholarship of teaching about policy requires engagement. Engagement requires that faculty invest their time and intellectual resources. Engagement requires thinking about critical social issues, pursuing relevant research, and developing relationships with policy makers and advocates. Without some engagement in policy issues, it is unlikely that faculty can effectively teach about policy and its many dimensions.

Once faculty persons are engaged in policy through the scholarship of discovery, integration, or application, their teaching will expand to include policy issues. The rich stories, failures, and successes that arise from work in the policy arena will find their way into the classroom as case studies and illustrations. Relationships with policy makers, clients, and advocates can lead to students' participation in research, field study, and policy conferences. These relationships may also lead policy makers and others back into the university as students or lecturers. The scholarship of teaching will enrich, and be enriched by, faculty's engagement in public policy.

FINDING WAYS TO ENGAGE

The scholarship of discovery, integration, application, and teaching can advance the well-being of our society but only if our intellectual and professional resources are invested to address the priority needs of individuals and families across the life-span. Each faculty person must choose how, and how much, to be involved in such policy related issues.

Not every faculty person will be equally involved in all aspects of policy engagement. Some will focus on discovery of new knowledge through research. Other faculty will focus on integration of ideas and communication with other scholars and students through professional publications and review books (see for example, the many volumes cited throughout this chapter). A segment of faculty will be more comfortable with direct communication with legislators and other decision-makers, while others will emphasize teaching roles.

Ideally, teams of faculty will form around policy issues and build on the best skills of each member. Teams may be able to face best the challenges of work that is applied, interdisciplinary, and integrative. It is no accident that many of the growing number of books on applied developmental science are co-authored, edited or reflect other forms of collaboration.

When faculty persons find *their* way to be engaged in policy, their work and lives will be challenged and enriched. Reciprocally, they will greatly enrich the policies that influence children, youth, and families.

REFERENCES

Aldous, J. & Dumon, W. (1991). Family policy in the 1980s. In A. Booth (Ed.), *Contemporary families: Looking forward, looking back*, (pp. 466-481). St. Paul, MN: National Council on Family Relations.

Anderson, E. & Skinner, D. (1995). The components of family policy education. *Journal of Family and Economics Issues, 16*(1), 65-77.

Bane, M. & Ellwood, D. (1994). *Welfare realities: From rhetoric to reform*. Cambridge, MA: Harvard University Press.

Biegel, D., Sales, E. & Schulz, R. (1991). *Family caregiving in chronic illness*. Thousand Oaks, CA: Sage.

Bogenschneider, K. (1995). Roles for professionals in building family policy: A case study of state family policy impact seminars. *Family Relations, 44*, 5-12.

Boyer, E. (1990). *Scholarship reconsidered: Priorities in the professorate*. Princeton, NJ: The Carnegie Foundation for the Advancement of Teaching.

Boyle, P. & Mulcahy, S. (1993). Public policy education. *Journal of Extension, 31*, 4-9.

Brooks-Gunn, J., Duncan, G. & Aber, L. (1997). *Neighborhood poverty: Context and consequences for children*. New York: Russell-Sage Foundation.

Chase-Lansdale, D. & Brooks-Gunn, J. (1996). Correlates of teen pregnancy and parenthood. In C. Fisher & R. Lerner (Eds.), *Applied developmental psychology*, (pp. 207-236). New York: McGraw-Hill.

Cole, E. & Duva, J. (1990). *Family preservation*. Chicago: Children's Welfare League of America.

Coontz, S. (1992). *The way we never were: American families and the nostalgia trap*. New York: Basic Books.

Coyne, A. (1993). Evaluating public policy: The administrative role. *International Journal of Public Administration, 16*, 1265-1284.

Cubbins, L. (1992). *Staying off public assistance: What enables a woman to stay off assistance once she has left?* Olympia, WA: Evergreen State College, Washington State Institute for Public Policy.

Duncan, G. & Brooks-Gunn, J. (1997). *The consequences of growing up poor*. New York: Russell-Sage Foundation.

Durlak, J. & Lipsey, M. (1991). A practitioner's guide to meta-analysis. *American Journal of Community Psychology, 19*, 291-332.

Ellwood, D. (1988). *Poor support: Poverty in the American family*. New York: Basic Books.

Fine, M. (1992). Families in the United States: Their current status and future prospects. *Family Relations, 41*, 430-435.

Fisher, C. (1993). The national conference on graduate education in the application of developmental science across the lifespan. *Journal of Applied Developmental Psychology, 14*, 1-10.

Franklin, C., Grant, D., Corcoran, J., Miller, P. & Bultman, L. (1997). Effectiveness of prevention programs for adolescent pregnancy: A meta-analysis. *Journal of Marriage and Family, 3*, 551-567.

Funiciello, T. (1993). *Tyranny of kindness: Dismantling the welfare system to end poverty in America.* New York: Atlantic Monthly Press.

Gelles, R. & Conte, J. (1991). Domestic violence and sexual abuse of children. In A. Booth (Ed.), *Contemporary families: Looking forward, looking back*, (pp. 327-340). St. Paul, MN: National Council on Family Relations.

Goetz, K. & Peck, S. (1994). *The basics of family support: A guide for state planners and others.* Chicago, IL: National Resource Center for Family Support Programs, Family Resource Coalition.

Gove, S. & Knott, J. (April, 1994). Can research agendas be developed to serve both academic and applied needs? *Opportunity and responsibility: The Link between public universities and state capitals.* Sacramento: California State University.

Hardy, J. & Zabin, L. (1991). *Adolescent pregnancy in an urban environment: Issues, programs, and evaluation.* Washington, DC: Urban Institute Press.

Hare, J., Gregorson, C., Pratt, C., Campbell, C., Kliewer, D. & Bruce, J. (1994). *Ballot Measure 16: The Death with Dignity Act. EM 8569.* Corvallis, OR: Oregon State University Extension Service Publications.

Haskins, R. (1993). Research and the political process. In G. Hendershot & F. LeClere (Eds.), *Family health: From data to policy*, (pp 61-63). St. Paul, MN: National Council on Family Relations.

Hawkins, J., Catalano, R. & Miller, J. (1992). Risk and protective factors for alcohol and other drug problems in adolescence and early adulthood: Implications for substance abuse prevention. *Psychological Bulletin, 112*, 64-105.

Jorgensen, S., Potts, V. & Camp, B. (1993). Project Taking Charge: Six month follow-up of a pregnancy prevention program for early adolescents. *Family Relations, 42*, 401-406.

Kagan, S. & Weissbourd, B. (1994). *Putting families first: America's family support movement and the challenge of change.* San Francisco, CA: Jossey-Bass.

Lerner, R. M. & Fisher, C. B. (1994). From applied developmental psychology to applied developmental science: Community coalitions and collaborative careers. In C. B. Fisher & R. M. Lerner (Eds.) *Applied developmental psychology* (pp. 505-522). New York: McGraw-Hill.

Lindbloom, C. & Woodhouse, E. (1993). *The policy-making process.* Englewood Cliffs, NJ: Prentice-Hall.

Lipsey, M. (1992). Juvenile delinquency treatment: A meta-analysis. In T. D. Cook, H. Cooper, D. Cordray, H. Hartman, L. Hedges, R. Light, T. Louis & F. Moesteller (Eds.), *Meta-analysis for explanation: A casebook*, (pp. 83-127). NY: Russell-Sage.

Lipsey, M. & Wilson, D. (1993). The efficacy of psychological, educational, and behavioral treatment: Confirmation from meta-analysis. *American Psychologist, 48*, 1181-1209.

Miller, B. & Moore, K. (1991). Adolescent sexual behavior, pregnancy, and parenting. In A. Booth (Ed.), *Contemporary families: Looking forward, looking back*, (pp. 307-326). St. Paul, MN: National Council on Family Relations.

Mishel, L. & Bernstein, J. (1993). *The state of working America: 1992-93.* Armonk, NY: M.E. Sharpe.

Monroe, P. (1987). Adolescent pregnancy legislation: The application of an analytic framework. *Family Relations, 36*, 15-21.

Monroe, P. (1991). Participation in state legislative activities: A practical guide for family scientists. *Family Relations, 40*, 324-331.

National Conference of State Legislatures. (1998). *Children, youth, and family issues: 1997 State Legislative Summary.* Washington, DC: National Conference of State Legislatures.

Olson, D. & Hanson, M. (1990). *NCFR Presidential Report 2001: Preparing families for the future.* St. Paul, MN: National Council on Family Relations.

Ooms, T. (1993). Implications of family health and family data on policy. In G. Hendershot & F. LeClere, (Eds.), *Family health: From data to policy*, (pp. 102-106). St. Paul, MN: National Council on Family Relations.

Ooms, T. & Weintaub, J. (1992). *Reducing family poverty: Tax-based and child support strategies.* Washington, DC: Family Impact Seminar.

Ooms, T., Cohen, E. & Hutchins, J. (1995). *Disconnected dads: Strategies for promoting responsible fatherhood.* Washington, DC: Family Impact Seminar.

Pentz, M. (1996). Primary prevention of adolescent drug abuse. In C. Fisher & R. Lerner (Eds.), *Applied developmental psychology*, (pp. 435-474). New York: McGraw-Hill.

Pratt, C. (1995). Family professionals and family policy: Strategies for influence. *Family Relations, 44*, 56-62.

Pratt, C., Katzev, A., Henderson, T. & Ozretich, R. (1997). *Building results: From wellness goals to positive outcomes for Oregon's children, youth, and families.* Salem, OR: Oregon Commission on Children and Families.

Premier's Council in Support of Alberta Families. (1993). *A family policy framework for the Province of Alberta.* Edmonton, Alberta, Canada: Author.

Rich, R. (1979). *Translating evaluation into policy.* Thousand Oaks, CA: Sage.

Rodman, H. & Sidden, J. (1992). A critique of pessimistic views about U.S. families. *Family Relations, 41*, 436-439.

Shadish, W., Cook, T. & Leviton, L. (1991). *Foundations of program evaluation: Theories of practice.* Thousand Oaks, CA: Sage.

Skinner, D. & Anderson, E. (1993). *Teaching family policy: A handbook of course syllabi, teaching strategies, and resources.* Minneapolis, MN: National Council on Family Relations.

Sprey, J. (1991). Current theorizing on the family. In A. Booth (Ed.), *Contemporary families: Looking forward, looking back,* (pp. 12-26). St. Paul, MN: National Council on Family Relations.

Stevens, G. (1992). *How to impact public policy for families.* Lincoln, NE: University of Nebraska-Lincoln, Cooperative Extension Service.

Trister, M. & Weill, J. (1991). *An advocate's guide to lobbying and political activity for non-profits.* Washington, DC: Children's Defense Fund.

Unrau, Y. (1994). Expanding the role of program evaluation in social welfare policy analysis. *Evaluation Review, 17*, 653-664.

U.S. House Select Sub-Committee on Children, Youth, & Families. (1986). *A strategy for strengthening families: Using family criteria in policymaking and program evaluation.* Washington, DC: U.S. Government Printing Office.

Webster, C., Hu, S. & Weeks, G. (1993). *Pathways to employment.* Olympia, WA: Evergreen State College, Washington State Institute for Public Policy.

Weissbourd, B. (1994). The evolution of the family resource movement. In S. Kagan & B. Weissbourd (Eds.), *Putting families first: America's family support movement and the challenge of change,* (pp. 28-48). San Francisco, CA: Jossey-Bass.

Wisensale, S. (1992). Toward the 21st century: Family change and public policy. *Family Relations, 41*, 417-422.

Wright, S. (1998). *Utah sourcebook on aging.* Salt Lake City, UT: University of Utah Gerontology Center.

Yoshikawa, H. (1994). Prevention as cumulative protection: Effects of early family support and education on chronic delinquency and its risks. *Psychological Bulletin, 115*, 28-54.

Zabin, L. & Hayward, S. (1993). *Adolescent sexual behavior and child-bearing.* Newbury Park, CA: Sage.

Zimmerman, S. (1992a). *Family policies and family well-being: The role of political culture.* Thousand Oaks, CA: Sage.

Zimmerman, S. (1992b). Family trends: What implications for family policy? *Family Relations, 41*, 423-429.

Implementing Public Policy Education:
The Role of the School or College

Charles McClintock, *Cornell University*

What is the role of the school or college within the larger university setting in implementing policy studies in applied developmental science? The answer to this question largely depends on whether academic critical mass lies within or across college boundaries, and if within, determining whether it cuts across departmental lines. Critical mass refers to the depth of expertise in public policy analysis and program management among the disciplines and fields of developmental science.

The college of today faces one or more of the following options—to focus developmental science policy expertise in a single department, to support a center or institute that links research and outreach efforts of faculty from several related departments, or to foster a "virtual department" by formalizing strong lateral ties for teaching, research and outreach across departmental and/or college units.[1] While the last direction is the least typical given that autonomous academic units form the building blocks of educational organizations (Weick, 1976), any of the choices requires attention to five aspects of change in higher education: 1) academic planning with vision, 2) sensitivity to the broader context, 3) faculty buy-in, 4) administrative "muscle," and 5) organizational climate.

These five issues provide a conceptual framework within which to examine the college's role in fostering policy studies in applied developmental science. The framework is drawn from research on organizational change (Cohen, March & Olsen, 1972; Kotter, 1996), the professoriate as a profession (Bess, 1998) and academic governance (Hofstadter, 1996). The evidence and analysis is based on a personal recounting of the creation of a new academic department, Policy Analysis and Management (PAM), in Cornell University's College of Human Ecology (McClintock, 1996). The academic focus of PAM is on policy analysis and program management in relation to family/social welfare, health care and consumer economics. The department includes undergraduate and graduate education, along with research and programmatic outreach functions. The faculty and staff for PAM were drawn from a merger of two existing departments: Consumer Economics and Housing that emphasized family and consumer policy issues, and Human Service Studies that concentrated on management, delivery and evaluation of health and human services.[2]

By nature, case studies are descriptive of specific situations but ideally with lessons that can be adapted for use elsewhere. The organization of applied developmental science has many variations across institutions nationally and the role of the college will differ somewhat depending on local conditions. For example, while PAM is concerned with child and family policy, a related concentration of expertise in applied developmental science at Cornell resides in a separate unit within the college: the Department of Human Development. Strengthening ties between PAM and the Department of Human Development around common policy interests is an important college goal. Instead of considering a merger of parts of these two departments, however, the College of Human Ecology supports two research and outreach units, the Bronfenbrenner Life

Course Center and the Family Life Development Center, to encourage individual and cross-departmental efforts in applied developmental science. These particular configurations at Cornell highlight the fact that, as with any case study, there are situational factors that limit generalizability across settings. For this reason, the five part conceptual framework is offered as a means of applying the lessons learned in creating a new policy department such as PAM to other colleges and universities.

FIVE ASPECTS OF CHANGE

Fostering lasting and effective structural change in organizations is rarely simple. In higher education, where administrative influence resides in trust and can be negated through the power of a resistant professoriate or student body, educationally effective decisions are vested in a positive *relationship* among faculty, administrators, and ultimately students who will vote with their feet on the attractiveness of new programs. Hence, no single stakeholder group has control over the process (Gitlow, 1995).

Implementing change also must be tempered by the distinctive dynamics of academia. Higher education exemplifies the two contradictory functions of most educational organizations: 1) a conservational role in preserving knowledge and imparting consistent intellectual, disciplinary and professional skills; and 2) a transformational role, which as Shils (1992) puts it, sets universities apart as the only societal institution that we can look to for "a transfigured existence." Hence, the role of the college in fostering change must always balance and nurture these opposing functions.

Academic Planning with Vision

Guskin (1996) emphasizes the importance of an energizing, distinctive, and briefly stated vision to discipline the often lengthy and wandering implementation process that follows a restructuring decision. Adaptation may be necessary during implementation but it must reinforce a vision that continues to chart the original direction and is viewed clearly as an improvement on what currently exists.

The academic vision that was developed by the steering committee for creating this new department was intended to be forward-looking and to join two scholarly approaches that typically are in separate units—the perspective of policy analysis and that of policy implementation (Averch & Dluhy, 1992; McClintock, 1996). In this context, policy analysis is represented by statistical modeling that examines the relative influence of a variety of causal factors on some outcome of interest, while policy implementation is concerned with the management, planning, delivery and evaluation of organizations and programs in their community, social and political contexts.

For example, in studying nonmarital births among adolescents, a policy analysis approach might use national probability sample data to examine the relative influence on birthrates of adolescents' future expectations, poverty and employment opportunities, peers, access to family planning services, and educational opportunities (Haveman, Wolfe, Wilson & Peterson, 1997). Policy implementation might focus on the design, delivery and management of pregnancy prevention programs and involve a variety of qualitative and quantitative evaluation methods to better understand the complex dynamics of intervening in the problem (Kirby, 1997). Both approaches are necessary yet insufficient by themselves to deal with the complexities of public policy formulation (Lindbloom & Woodhouse, 1993; McClintock & Colosi, 1998).

A critical part of shaping the vision for PAM was to create something new, not just a merger of two existing units, that addressed an academic frontier or goal toward which faculty could strive over a long time frame. Developing a vision leads to consideration of a second aspect of the conceptual frameworks: the academic and policy contexts within which educational change occurs.

Sensitivity to Broader Context

The role of the college with regard to context is to ensure that faculty examine policy programs at other campuses, identify key professional associations in which to participate, and understand the policy environment—all of which are crucial to developing a distinctive program identity. An analysis of context helps to define an academic niche that gives distinctive purpose and insures sources of external support to the department, as well as means of comparing or ranking performance with competitor programs. The College of Human Ecology met this need by supporting faculty travel to other institutions to gather first-hand impressions, reviewing program and curriculum materials from a wide range of peer institution policy programs, especially including those within New York State, and funding a graduate assistant to examine empirical literature on these issues (see, for example, Averch & Dluhy, 1992).

The result of this analysis led the steering committee to identify a primary professional association, the Association of Public Policy Analysis and Management (APPAM), as a focal point for comparing the new department to other policy departments and schools. At the same time, it was recognized that faculty would continue to participate in a variety of professional groups relevant to their particular research areas, including applied economics, program evaluation, social work, and family and consumer sciences. In applied developmental science there is a similar range of professional associations and meetings in child development, family and consumer sciences, and human sciences that might be appropriate, as well as innovative frameworks and journals for emphasizing the cross-cutting mission and settings of this emerging academic area (see, for example, Lerner, Fisher & Weinberg, 1997).

The public policy context was another important consideration in developing the academic plan for PAM. American public policy and management are strongly shaped by the federalist intergovernmental structure in which authority and accountability are shared across national, state and local government. Currently, the devolution shift from national to state and community levels of governance known as the "new federalism" is exemplified by welfare reform (McClintock & Colosi, 1998). The privatization of many heretofore public health functions through managed care is another critical policy focus for applied developmental science in the foreseeable future. In addition, the private nonprofit sector plays a significant role in funding and delivering human services, and the role of community groups, volunteers and consumers is critical to the effectiveness of policy formulation, analysis and implementation.

Forward-looking academic programs will emphasize these aspects of the heterogeneous policy context, as well as relationship of public and private services to informal family, neighborhood and community resources, and asset-based perspectives on human development and family studies (see, for example, Benson, Leffert, Scales & Blyth, 1998). One role for the college in this process is to ensure that faculty are exposed to the work of leading academics and public policy practitioners through cross-disciplinary visiting scholar and speaker programs.

College of Human Ecology support of policy outreach for faculty scholarship is also helpful in order to highlight the value of research to practitioners as well as influence faculty choice of research topics that will be relevant to policy needs. These goals were supported by the college through initiation of a policy seminar series for state and community leaders (McClintock, 1999). Each of these efforts to increase awareness of context was helpful in assisting with the third factor in the conceptual framework: faculty buy-in.

Faculty Buy-in

The two groups represented in PAM's academic plan—those involved with policy analysis and with policy implementation—often have diverging views, epistemologies, methodologies, values, disciplinary backgrounds, and work cultures. For these reasons, they typically work in separate departments or schools and joining them in the same unit is a challenge.[3] Because of these differences, it was critical that the vision for PAM include both groups as two essential sides of the same coin. It will remain a leadership challenge to engage the two groups in productive collaboration, yet it is worth noting that contrasting professional cultures in an organization can maintain diversity of expertise and responsiveness to unanticipated academic and policy contexts that inevitably occur over time (Weick, 1977).

Top-down change occurs on many campuses but, similar to numerous corporate mergers that are directed solely by upper management, may have limited success due to implementation problems among those employees who are expected to do the work. This situation can be avoided, even with change initiated at the top, by creating mechanisms for learning, adaptation and productive political process among faculty, students, staff and the outside communities who rely on academic contributions (Stacey, 1992).

The process of engaging faculty in change was greatly assisted by the two department chairs who met weekly and had regular discussions of the possibilities at department meetings. These early meetings focused on areas in which the departments could easily merge administrative and decision-making structures. Emphasizing administrative matters at this stage was a way of psychologically preparing faculty for some of the difficult academic program choices that eventually needed to be made. After about one semester of these initial discussions, a formal steering committee was established with faculty from the two departments as well as from other units with policy interests, to prepare an academic plan for a new department.

A critical aspect of faculty buy-in was resource flexibility. Following several years of reductions in state budgets, it was critical for the faculty to have a sense that there would be sufficient resources available to make the new department a success. The role of the College of Human Ecology was to hold open faculty lines that had been vacated over several years in order to offer the opportunity for infusing PAM with fresh professorial faces including that of a senior appointment for department chair with a national reputation for strong academic leadership in policy. There was also a commitment to faculty development in the new department, especially in relation to insuring quality in the teaching program and its representation of the policy analyst and policy implementor perspectives for students.

The steering committee produced a merger plan within four months that was decisively supported by departmental and college faculty. During the ensuing academic year, various joint committees were formed to develop important specifics about curriculum, outreach programs, tenure and promotion procedures, governance, and administrative organization, and in the semester prior to the official merger, the two faculties met together for all departmental meetings.

Not all faculty from the two merging departments were equally enthusiastic about the academic plan, and it is possible that in a few instances the change hastened a retirement or departure for a different campus. However, the various merger implementation committees provided opportunities for faculty involvement which enhanced buy-in on the part of the vast majority of those directly affected. A parallel process of regular meetings, involvement and input was established for administrative staff in the two departments. There were no layoffs as a result of the merger although some reduction in administrative resources was achieved through natural attrition. The College of Human Ecology was very supportive of addressing serious concerns about the implications of the merger on the part of staff who too often are an afterthought in the status hierarchy of academia.

Administrative "Muscle"

Perhaps this term seems out of place since in a collegial organization such as the university where decision-making based on hierarchical authority alone is not likely to produce quality change. Nevertheless, while hoping for consensus on critical issues, college administrators must be prepared to make choices in the absence of agreement among faculty or students. Turf wars are common in academia and there were various skirmishes along the road to merger that presented complex differences of opinion where it was necessary for the college to offer incentives, set boundaries and make choices.

First, as noted earlier, the two department chairs began to meet regularly which helped bring faculty along in the change process. These meetings were stimulated, however, by the college's position that additional budget cuts from the state would be applied to each of the two units, further hampering current programs. The incentive of retaining frozen positions for a reconfigured department was critical for motivating faculty to re-think their specialty areas.

Second, once the idea of a merger was accepted, it was important to give the steering committee an ambitious goal and time frame to avoid the problem of a long process leading to fractionation and a report that tried to please all. The goal was to create change and join together different groups into something new, and this required a very specific charge to the steering committee with a firm due date for a product. Allowing for summer break, the original one semester time frame for preparing and voting on an academic plan was missed only by a month. As it turned out, the summer break allowed for time to gather reactions to the academic plan from faculty and administrators around the campus, a process that provided additional support for the vision. The role of the college was to push the steering committee to produce an academic plan on schedule so that the broader faculty groups could discuss and eventually vote on it.

Third, disciplinary battles are among the most intense in academia and the creation of a policy department is likely to bring them to the fore, since policy studies typically cut across disciplines. Similar to each department in the College of Human Ecology, PAM is an interdisciplinary unit representing economics, psychology, sociology, family and consumer sciences, education and social work. One of the tensions in the plan was the role of economics and statistics in the required core for undergraduates. The economists argued for the centrality of their comparatively unified conceptual and statistical tools in policy analysis, while others noted the educational value of multiple perspectives and methods for understanding the complex interplay of psychological, social, and political factors in policy formulation and implementation.

Ultimately this issue was resolved by the dean who endorsed one of two alternate curriculum plans that, in addition to two economics and three research methods/statistics courses, included broad introductory courses in policy analysis and in non-profit management, as well as a sophomore level course called Critical Perspectives. This latter course was designed to educate students about different ways of creating knowledge and analyzing the policy world, including the political and value perspectives inherent in any particular approach to policy analysis and management. Another advantage of having a final decision on the undergraduate curriculum was that it gave the faculty a concrete picture of how the department would evolve in the future. This specificity is often missing in organizational change efforts in which conflict is temporarily avoided through broad rhetoric that allows different groups to interpret plans through their respective but differing desires.

A final difficult issue was whether to retain an accredited undergraduate social work program with its externally determined requirements including intensively supervised field work. Social work strongly represents the program implementation side of the department with its emphasis on human service delivery in the context of individual, group, organizational, community, and policy issues, yet it was not clear in the minds of a majority of faculty that the program would enroll enough students to justify the cost. Personnel shifts in the social work program added uncertainty to its leadership and, after a long period of committee review and faculty debate, the dean of the College of Human Ecology accepted the majority faculty view not to continue the program. At the same time, in parallel with an honors research program, the faculty endorsed an honors program in experiential learning in which students emphasize first-hand exposure to professional practices in human service policy analysis and management. This honors program extends the college's long-standing support for field study (McClintock & Beck, 1998).

Organizational Climate

College administrators always need to be sensitive to climate as a key aspect of the context of change. At Cornell, the time was ripe for the creation of a new academic department in the social and health policy arena that would strengthen academic programs and provide some modest administrative savings since the university had just recruited a new president who identified cross-unit "synergy" as one of his goals. Interest was also being expressed in strengthening the social sciences at Cornell. These two events created a vacuum which the college stepped into quickly in order to have as much influence as possible over the shape of its own policy programs.

The two constituent units merging into the new department of Policy Analysis and Management were about to undergo their own U.S. Department of Agriculture program reviews. These reviews, which were postponed by the college due to the merger, were coming after a period of nearly seven years of budget reductions from the state in which faculty lines and support services had been lost. The combination of annual budget reductions and an impending external program review created an atmosphere conducive to significant structural change. Working with the department chairs and faculty, the college tried to establish the principle that restructuring was the best way to maintain quality and maximize local influence over the shape of a new direction. Also, by creating the steering committee for planning, the college was able to provide an action venue for many faculty who had long expressed the need for greater emphasis on policy and management.

A final aspect of the organizational climate related to Cornell University's decentralized structure for budgeting and governance in which colleges enjoy considerable academic autonomy. As mentioned earlier, having sufficient control over resources to hire new faculty in a merged department was a major factor in giving faculty a sense that they could shape their academic destiny. Without resource flexibility, the organizational climate and resulting faculty energy for change might have been more resistant.

ORGANIZATIONAL LEARNING AND ADAPTABILITY

The capacity for learning and adaptability, rather than any particular adaptive form, is key to understanding how organizations survive or become extinct (Weick, 1977). This idea is central to dynamic systems and chaos theory concepts which highlight the role of small unanticipated changes that amplify in positive reinforcement cycles over time into large and powerful forces (Stacey, 1992). In the setting of academic change, these ideas lead to a role for the college and its academic administration that de-emphasizes control and values learning, self-organizing teams, diversity in organizational culture, and sufficient resources for experimentation and risk taking in new ventures (Guskin, 1996).

An emphasis on control is also likely to overlook the role of chance in successful outcomes. As noted by Cohen, March and Olsen (1972) in their analysis of organizational decision-making, many "choices" are the result of independent streams of people, their attention span, and problems and solutions which randomly flow together creating opportunistic connections. Chance alone often highlights a subgroup's favored solution which gets attached to a pressing problem that then captures the attention of those people who happen to be present in the situation. While this rendering of decision-making downplays intentionality a bit too much, retrospective interpretations of events also convey an unjustified rationality to stochastic processes as well as overemphasizing decision maker credit for success and externalized blame for failure. It would be naive to think that a change strategy only emphasizing planning and control could produce the positive outcome of a strongly endorsed merger. For instance, it was partly serendipitous that there was no opposition from other policy and management-oriented programs across the campus, and, indeed, strong support for the new department from university administration. This situation might well have been less supportive at a campus with more centralized academic planning or during another time at Cornell.

Given that all events cannot be controlled, what is the role of the college in promoting needed change? The answer from this case study suggests a role for administrators that creates the *conditions* for ongoing learning about academic effectiveness, as well as productive conflict among the various campus and off-campus groups who have a stake or interest in academic programs in applied developmental science. Such a role is particularly important for this area of scholarship whose evolution is tied to the interplay between society and the academy around new knowledge in human development, and related policy developments in areas such as welfare reform, early childhood education, and health care.

Perhaps it is permissible to end a brief case study exposition such as this with popular quotes that sum up two final lessons for the role of the college in implementing policy education in applied developmental science. The first, from entertainer Bill Cosby, emphasizes the need for vision and decisiveness and the second, from hockey star Wayne Gretzky, reminds us of the need to pursue important goals no matter what the odds:

> "I don't know the key to success, but the key to failure is trying to please everybody." Bill Cosby

"One hundred percent of the shots you don't take don't go in."
Wayne Gretzky

NOTES

Thanks are due to Keith Bryant, Francille M. Firebaugh, Jenny Gerner and John Murray for helpful comments in revising this chapter.

1. Even if the single department choice is made, there is a strong likelihood in the multidisciplinary policy arena that ties with other units will be desirable and necessary for creating academic strength that draws on complementary expertise across departments.

2. Each department had changed its name since the college's reorganization in 1968. Until the early 1980s, Consumer Economics and Housing had been named Consumer Economics and Public Policy, reflecting a long-standing policy analysis focus. At about the same time, the Department of Community Service Education changed its name to Human Service Studies expanding from an emphasis on community services to state and federal policy implementation, planning and evaluation.

3. Until the mid-1980s, the two departments shared an interdepartmental major, Policy Analysis and Social Planning, and its name reflected these two orientations. The program fell victim to a dominant dynamic of higher education; the two faculties moved toward their respective specializations and could not agree by themselves on a common undergraduate curriculum. At that time, the college had not played a forceful role in preserving this interdepartmental effort.

REFERENCES

Averch, H. & Dluhy, M. (1992). Teaching public administration, public management, and policy analysis: Convergence or divergence in the masters core. *Journal of Policy Analysis and Management, 11*, 541-551.

Benson, P. L., Leffert, N., Scales, P. C. & Blyth, D. A. (1998). Beyond the "village" rhetoric: Creating healthy communities for children and adolescents. *Applied Developmental Science, 2*(3), 138-159.

Bess, J. L. (1998). Contract systems, bureaucracies, and faculty motivation: The probable effects of a no-tenure policy. *Journal of Higher Education, 69*, 1-23.

Cohen, M. D., March, J. G. & Olsen, J. P. (1972). A garbage can model of organizational choice. *Administrative Science Quarterly, 17*, 1-25.

Gitlow, A. (1995). *Reflections on higher education: A dean's view.* New York: University Press of America.

Guskin, A. E. (1996). Facing the future: The change process in restructuring universities. *Change, 28*, 27-37.

Haveman, R., Wolfe, B., Wilson, K. & Peterson, E. (1997). Do teens make rational choices?: The case of teen nonmarital childbearing. Institute for Research on Poverty, Paper # 1137-97. Madison, WI: University of Wisconsin-Madison.

Hofstadter, R. (1996). *Academic freedom in the age of the college.* New Brunswick, NJ: Transaction Publishers.

Kirby, D. (1997). No easy answers: Research findings on programs to reduce teen pregnancy. Washington, DC: National Campaign to Prevent Teen Pregnancy, Task Force on Effective Programs and Research.

Kotter, J. P. (1996). *Leading change.* Boston, MA: Harvard Business School Press.

Lerner, R. M., Fisher, C. B. & Weinberg, R. A. (1997). Applied developmental science: Scholarship for our times. *Applied Developmental Science, 1*, 2-3.

Lindbloom, C. E. & Woodhouse, E. J. (1993). *The policy-making process.* New Jersey: Prentice-Hall.

McClintock, C. (1996). *Academic plan for the creation of the department of policy analysis and management in the College of Human Ecology, Cornell University* (pp. 269-274). Ithaca, NY: Cornell University.

McClintock, C. (1999). Policy seminars for state and community leaders. In T. Chibucos & R. Lerner (Eds.) *Serving children and families through community-university partnerships: Success stories.* Norwell, MA: Kluwer.

McClintock, C. & Beck, S. (1998). Multicultural education in urban affairs: Field-based learning about diversity. *Journal of Family and Consumer Sciences, 90*(1), 49-53.

McClintock, C. & Colosi, L. (1998). Evaluating welfare reform: A framework for including the urgent and the important. *Evaluation Review, 22*, 668-694.

Shils, E. A. (1992). The universities, the social sciences and liberal democracy. *Interchange, 23*, 183-223.

Stacey, R. D. (1992). *Managing the unknowable: Strategic boundaries between order and chaos in organizations.* San Francisco, CA: Jossey-Bass.

Weick, K. E. (1976). Educational organizations as loosely coupled systems. *Administrative Science Quarterly, 21*, 1-19.

Implementing Public Policy Education:
The Role of the University
James C. Votruba, *Northern Kentucky University*

As exemplified by the exchanges at the Third National Applied Developmental Science Conference, I believe that applied developmental science (ADS) is providing the intellectual foundation for the twenty-first century university; it is an intellectual foundation that emphasizes both scholarly excellence and public engagement. ADS scholars are positioned to help shape the twenty-first century university. The purpose of this chapter is to discuss the challenges that we must confront if we are to build universities in which ADS can thrive.

In his last published essay, Ernest Boyer (1996) wrote, "The academy must become a more vigorous partner in the search for answers to our most pressing social, civic, economic, and moral problems and must reaffirm its historic commitment to the scholarship of engagement" (p. 11). It is the scholarship of engagement that ADS is all about. ADS reaffirms the special covenant that has historically existed between American higher education and the public whom we serve; a covenant that has resulted in enormous benefit both to society and the academy. In an age of increasing public skepticism regarding the willingness and capacity of universities to impact our most pressing social concerns, ADS provides both a vision and strategy for the scholarship of engagement. The challenge that we confront is to translate that vision into reality.

Over the past eight years, my work at Michigan State and now at Northern Kentucky University, as well as with a large and diverse array of universities across the nation, has focused on how we can create institutional environments that support the scholarship of engagement. I want to focus on what I believe to be the key challenges that must be addressed if the scholarship of engagement is to become deeply imbedded in our universities.

The first challenge is to reconceptualize our fundamental academic mission. Traditionally, universities have described their mission as involving teaching, research, and service with each treated as a conceptually distinct form of professional activity. The scholarship of engagement challenges this formulation. If I and several of my graduate and undergraduate students are involved in a collaborative research project with a local community-based health organization designed to help understand better the problem of infant mortality among low income families, is this research, teaching, or service? The answer is that it is all three. If universities are going to be supportive of the scholarship of engagement, they must begin by blurring the distinction between what is research, teaching, and service and recognize that these mission dimensions are more seamless than we have previously acknowledged. The twenty-first century university will formulate its mission around a set of knowledge-based activities that mutually reinforce and support one another and contribute to our central purpose to discover, transmit, and apply knowledge.

Reformulating our mission has enormous consequences for how we value certain forms of faculty professional activity. For example, most of our campuses construct their promotion and tenure guidelines around the teaching, research, and

118

*Social Change, Public Policy, and Community Collaborations: Training
Human Development Professionals for the Twenty-First Century*

service trilogy. Because the scholarship of engagement cuts across all three mission dimensions, faculty members are confronted with the choice of how best to describe and position their work. If it is done in response to a community need, should they place it under the service category? Certainly it has a service dimension. But it also involves cutting-edge research. If universities are going to support the scholarship of engagement as represented by ADS, they must ensure that promotion and tenure criteria don't inadvertently force categorizations that result in diminishing a faculty member's work.

The second challenge that we must confront is to broaden the epistemological framework of the university to accommodate the scholarship of engagement. Referring to the scholarship of engagement, Donald Schön (1995) writes, "If the new scholarship is to mean anything, it must imply a kind of action research with norms of its own, which will conflict with the norms of technical-rationality—the prevailing epistemology built into the research universities" (p. 27). The point is that the research university is an institution built around a particular view of knowledge which our notions of the scholarship of engagement will inevitably challenge. Space does not permit a full explication of this argument. Suffice it to say that new forms of scholarship require a new epistemology if these new forms are to achieve academic legitimacy.

The third challenge is to demonstrate a deeper capacity for truly inter-disciplinary work. I believe that, on most of our campuses, we talk a better game than we do related to interdisciplinary scholarship. I must admit that I have not had very good luck getting interdisciplinary teams to engage in collaborative work. Even within the social sciences, disciplines speak different languages, build on different theory bases, enjoy differential status, and often evidence a form of academic hubris that precludes real collaboration. I believe that the university's capacity to influence both public policy and public programs in the area of human development requires that we strengthen our capacity to work across disciplines. Until we do so, we will limit our ability to impact complex policy and program decisions.

The fourth challenge is to deepen our understanding of how to create and sustain external partnerships. Michigan State University has recently created an ADS graduate specialization that involves approximately thirty active faculty from across a broad range of disciplines. MSU has developed a dozen or so outreach partnerships that are intended to be long term and involve a number of discreet scholarly projects that build on the intersection of faculty and graduate student interests with the needs of our partners. As these partnerships have expanded and matured, we have learned important lessons concerning "principles of good practice" related to university-community partnerships. We have learned that these collaborations are labor intensive, require constant nurturing, and are prone to serious miscommunication. We have also learned that the partnerships are aided by having very specific plans of work, negotiated products, clearly defined responsibilities, agreed upon timelines, shared resource commitments, and a strategy for disengagement when the partnership has run its course. The ADS national network provides a useful forum for exploring what other institutions have learned about partnership development in support of the scholarship of engagement.

The fifth challenge that we confront involves strengthening the university's faculty and the unit-level incentive and reward system to support the scholarship of engagement. Said another way, we need to "incentivize" the system on behalf of our work. It runs counter to the academic culture to assert that faculty must engage in one form of scholarship or another. However, leaders have it within their power to support those units and individuals who want to pursue the scholarship of engagement. They can do so for new projects, bridge funding to assist a unit to augment their personnel or programmatic resources, and evaluative standards that highlight the importance of the scholarship of engagement along with more traditional forms of scholarship.

The sixth challenge is to strengthen faculty development in support of the scholarship of engagement. If we are serious about institutionalizing our work, we cannot leave it to faculty members to intuit themselves into this new form of scholarship. Most faculty members leave their graduate programs with little or no experience in conducting scholarship in partnership with communities. Far too often they learn how to do this through trial and error. A few fortunate ones find themselves in departments where they receive mentoring from senior faculty who are experienced in collaborative work. What we have learned the hard way is that faculty who are successful in the scholarship of engagement require more than subject area competence. They must be sensitive to local cultures and values. They must have the ability to speak in terms that the public can understand. They must know how to establish and sustain trust. Most importantly, they must understand that, when they engage in community-based collaboration, they do so as both a teacher and learner with the community playing both roles as well. It is this willingness on the part of both the faculty and the community to be both teacher and learner that is the foundation on which the partnerships are built.

The seventh challenge that we confront is to incorporate the scholarship of engagement in the university's annual planning and budgeting process. Over the past several years, Michigan State has created the expectation that each academic unit will contribute to the full breadth of the academic mission including what we are referring to here as the scholarship of engagement. Units are budgeted to support the full breadth of the mission and held accountable for performance. Each year as part of the annual planning and evaluation process, units meet with the provost to review their accomplishments across the mission and to make the case for new resources based on plans that they have developed. As part of this process, the provost reviews what has been accomplished and what is planned related to community-based collaborative scholarship. Over the past eight years, MSU has reallocated approximately $35M, much of which has gone to support the outreach efforts of the campus including the scholarship of engagement. The point is that, if the university is to take seriously the scholarship of engagement, it must be supported by resources as well as rhetoric.

The eighth challenge is to create new organizational models that support the scholarship of engagement. One such strategy is to create new centers and institutes that promote collaborative community-based work. It was this approach that led to the creation of MSU's Institute for Children, Youth, and Families. In addition, several universities are experimenting with "virtual organizations" designed to bring together faculty around new and emerging issues that lend themselves to interdisciplinary problem-focused scholarship. In most cases, these efforts are supported by modest seed funding that can be used to leverage larger grants to support cutting-edge research and evaluation. In a more radical vein, a few universities are even considering the formation of separate 501(c)(3) organizations that are free of traditional bureaucratic drag and are able to respond quickly to new opportunities as they emerge. MSU has also created a new form of knowledge professional called a "linker" who serves to bridge the academic expertise of the faculty with the needs of the community. These linkers are professionals who move comfortably in both the university and the community and know how to relate each to the other. What I want to emphasize is that universities committed to the scholarship of engagement must create organizational systems to support this work.

The ninth challenge that I want to discuss is the need to promote institutional leadership on behalf of our work. There is no question that, for the scholarship of engagement to flourish, it must be supported at the highest levels of the university.

Those of us who are championing this work must pay careful attention to cultivating support from our governing boards, presidents, and provosts. However, it is equally important to have deans and chairs who both support this new arena of scholarship and are capable and willing to lead its development. Several years ago, Michigan State initiated a department chair leadership development program designed to help chairs lead across the full breadth of their unit's academic mission. This program has helped strengthen leadership on behalf of collaborative scholarship at the development level where it is most needed. We have also identified a few exemplar departments that were given a modest amount of additional resources to engage in strategic planning across the full breadth of their mission as well as the creation of a faculty evaluation system that is aligned with the strategic planning process.

The final challenge that I want to briefly mention is the need to organize strong and vocal external constituencies on behalf of our work. A close friend of mine in agricultural economics is quick to point out that the scholarship of engagement will never receive strong support until it has a well organized and powerful set of advocacy groups that help ensure that both the university and the public policy process are supportive of their needs. Is it possible to develop a similar set of advocacy groups on behalf of the collaborative work that universities conduct on behalf of children, youth, and family issues or health issues? I have struggled with this question and have found no good answer. However, I remain convinced that, until we do find an answer, the interests of those whom we are trying to serve and who most need our support will remain underserved.

As was clear at the Third National ADS Conference, we all have much for which we can be proud. The scholarship of engagement in general and applied developmental science in particular have struck a respondent cord among faculty across the nation. All ADS scholars should take credit for this development and feel energized to continue advancing the agenda. It is also true that the rhetoric of engagement is now on the lips of university presidents and provosts who have become advocates for greater involvement with issues of public concern. However, it is my experience that, far too often, this rhetoric is not being translated into well thought out strategies for addressing the challenges that I have described here. This is reinforced by the enormous disconnect that exists on many campuses between what senior administrative officers say they value and what is actually valued at the college and departmental level.

We need more institutional leaders who have the courage and commitment to address the challenges that impede the further development of the scholarship of engagement on each of our campuses. It is only through addressing these challenges that our universities will usher in a new era of scholarship that is characterized by both academic excellence and public engagement.

REFERENCES

Boyer, E. L. (1996). The scholarship of engagement. *Journal of Public Service and Outreach, 1*(1), 11-20.
Schön, D. A. (1995, November/December). Knowing-in-action: The new scholarship requires a new epistemology. *Change*, 27-34.

Funding Opportunities for Applied Developmental Science

Lonnie R. Sherrod, *William T. Grant Foundation*

This chapter addresses the private funding opportunities available—or that may be created—for research and training in applied developmental science. Applied developmental science, with its emphasis on university-community collaborations and on dissemination of research and training in applied science, creates a potential to revive philanthropy's interest in research in a way that has not happened since its origins at the turn of the century.

THE ORIGINS OF PHILANTHROPY

The industrialization of the early twentieth century created numerous self-made men committed to using their business skills as well as their accumulated wealth to heal some of the emerging social ills. These new philanthropists, such as Carnegie and Rockefeller, began their work in the context of a variety of charities and relief organizations. They saw these charities as providing temporary relief by treating symptoms; their goal, however, was to cure the core causes of social problems—to accomplish social change. This attitude arose in the private sector at a time when government was not involved in social welfare and reform. Hence, there was a clear role for the privately funded philanthropies. And several of the United State's largest and most influential foundations today arose early in this century: the Russell Sage Foundation in 1907, the Carnegie Corporation in 1911, the Rockefeller Foundation in 1913, and the Commonwealth Fund in 1918. As general purpose foundations, their objective was to advance public welfare, but science was seen as a means to that goal. Research in the social sciences, with its clear distinction between cause and effect, provided a strategy for approaching the solution of social ills, by identifying core causes of problems that could then be addressed, as opposed to alleviating symptoms or temporarily providing relief (Cahan, 1986; Katz & Katz, 1981). Although most of these new foundations did not provide substantial support directly for science, the appreciation of science as a tool provided a funding context that fueled the growth of the social behavioral sciences and the universities in which they became housed.

THE GROWTH OF PHILANTHROPY IN THE UNITED STATES

As was true a century ago, the globalization of market economies and the emergence of new technologies in communication and information processing have again fueled economic growth which has driven an increase in philanthropy in this country in recent decades. Private foundations by their nature are affluent, so they benefit from the same domestic economic policies that benefit business and affluent citizens. The tax laws in the U.S. create an incentive for individual charity and are an important factor in accounting for the growth of philanthropy in the U.S. relative to other parts of the world.

The last few decades have, in fact, been characterized by substantial growth both in the size of existing foundations, even after controlling for inflation, and in the number and types of foundations in the U.S. The number of private foundations in the U.S. has nearly doubled since the mid-1970s, and the total assets of these foundations have doubled even after considering the impact of inflation. The largest decade of growth was in the 1980s (28%), reflecting the economic boom of that decade, followed by the 1950s (22%) (Heimann, 1973; Renz & Lawrence, 1993). Since the 1960s foundations have been required by federal law to pay out a minimum percentage of their assets, currently 5%. Thus, as foundation resources grow so does their potential impact.

In addition to growing in absolute numbers and assets, foundations in the U.S. have become increasingly diverse. Four major types of foundations currently exist in the U.S. All of the foundations I have so far mentioned, including the William T. Grant Foundation, are *independent foundations*. They are intended to be self-perpetuating. They have a substantial endowment. The interest earned on this corpus supports programs and projects, according to the mission established by the founder. Most major independent foundations are governed by boards of directors that are largely independent of the founding family or corporate entity. There are three other types of foundations. Some foundations may be direct arms of the families or corporations that established them. In these cases, they function collaboratively with the founding family members or corporate boards. These are designed as *family or corporate foundations*. *Community foundations* have also arisen to serve the needs of specific communities. These foundations both receive contributions and dispense grant support. They are typically mandated to support only local programs—to contribute to the well-being of a designated community area, typically city, county or state. The final type of foundation is the *operating foundation*. Regardless of source of endowment or funding, these foundations actually develop and run the projects that they fund.

These "other" types of foundations have represented a substantial portion of the growth in the last decades. These newer types of foundations are now funding as much as, and in some areas more than, independent foundations. Predictions are that local philanthropic activities, such as community foundations, will represent the most intense area of future philanthropic activity (Hall, 1988; Nason, 1989).

The newer expansion of philanthropy has contributed little to the growth or development of the social sciences across the past couple of decades, in contrast to the role of philanthropy earlier in the century. Currently, only 2%-5% of both dollars and number of grants goes directly to science/technology or to social science. Corporate and community foundations are less likely to fund social science although they do fund relevant other categories, specifically education and human services which tend not to be research based (Renz & Lawrence, 1993).

THE SEPARATION OF PHILANTHROPY AND RESEARCH

The latter day growth of philanthropy in the U.S. has not been guided by the notion that propelled it during its origins earlier in the century: that science offers a useful means of addressing social problems. Foundations have, however, continued to search for ways of increasing their effectiveness in addressing social problems. With increasing frequency, social programs have been funded that adopt comprehensive approaches to problem solving rather than target specific issues. Collaborations of community constituencies have been encouraged or required. Community-wide initiatives have been developed. Collaborations of foundations have developed to share resources and wisdom. That is, a range of new strategies and targets has been sought by philanthropy in an effort to increase its effectiveness. Research has not, however, generally been seen to be very directly helpful in enhancing effectiveness except in looking to evaluation research methods to *demonstrate* effectiveness. And this look to evaluation has not even moved beyond this limited conception of demonstrating effectiveness to the broader view that I propose later in this chapter.

There are several possible explanations for the increasing separation of science support and philanthropy, and for the departure from the historical trends that characterized the early development of both fields. The first is the increased role of government, particularly at the federal level. There are now several governmental agencies whose primary mission is the support of research. Examples such as the National Science Foundation need not be described because they are all familiar to the scholars involved in applied developmental science. However, government at all levels, local as well as federal, has assumed a major role in *all* areas of philanthropic endeavors. In response to government's entry into social welfare efforts, philanthropy has redefined its role to identify a niche that distinguishes its efforts from those of government. Private funding gets things started with the idea that effective undertakings will then be sustained by government funding. This is perhaps a questionable expectation, particularly in these days when government is downsizing. However, the point is that governmental support for research does not fully explain philanthropy's abandonment of science as a tool in attempting social change because government has also increased its role in other areas, such as social welfare, where philanthropic activity has not decreased.

A second factor may be a perception that social conditions have deteriorated, particularly for children and families. As the urgency of social problems increases, research can come to be viewed as an unaffordable luxury, and directed efforts aimed at quick fixes sought. Children may be worse off than they were a few decades ago, and they certainly merit our help, but they do not live in poorer conditions than they did a century ago. In fact, recognizing society's views of children during the late nineteenth century (before child labor and juvenile justice laws were enacted), one may even argue that today's children enjoy a more privileged position. Nonetheless, at that time, philanthropists recognized that research is not a luxury; research of varied types was recognized to be necessary to the success of society. In fact, as social conditions worsen, research becomes more important in order to insure that resources aimed at improving social welfare are used wisely. Thus, this factor also cannot fully explain the separation of philanthropy and science.

Another factor may be that the social sciences have not lived up to their promise of usefulness. Prewitt (1995) emphasizes the importance of objectivity in the early development of the social sciences and refers to the potential of the social-behavioral sciences to serve as the "systematic social intelligence" of society. Advocacy and neutrality (or objectivity) have been viewed to conflict, but social science research integrates them by imparting objectivity to strategies aimed at the betterment of society. Knowledge rather than ideology determines the choice of solutions to social problems. It is this view of science that appealed to the early philanthropists and that needs to be emphasized by applied developmental science.

Some in philanthropy, perhaps especially in its newer forms, see wisdom, knowledge, or intelligence to reside in experience that is more firmly grounded in the "real world" than seems to be true for science. There are those who view science as relegated to universities which have become increasingly isolated from the communities in which they reside; the knowledge housed in universities is not viewed to relate to the problems addressed in the real world, outside the academy. Science has been seen to be reductionistic and not sufficiently complex to deal with the real world problems confronted by foundations in their daily work. And some philanthropists and others oriented to promoting the social good have developed their own forms of wisdom and knowledge based on experience.

Additionally many communities fear or resent research, seeking it as only taking from them without offering anything in return, and foundations have been sensitive to this view of community residents.

Applied developmental science has the potential to confront these views and to reaffirm the place of social science as the "systematic social intelligence" of society. It brings research out of the academy and demonstrates its usefulness in multiple ways. It educates and helps as well as generating new knowledge. It has the potential to rebuild the partnership between philanthropy and research. There are three relevant areas where funding may be pursued: university-community collaborations, dissemination of research to non-research audiences, and training in applied developmental science.

UNIVERSITY-COMMUNITY PARTNERSHIPS

Applied developmental science blurs the distinction between basic and applied research. All research is potentially applicable to social problems. Research differs in the time frame of that application and in the source of the research question, but neither factor undermines relevance to social problems. Research typically labeled "applied" has immediate relevance but can also yield basic knowledge, whereas "basic" research may become relevant in unexpected ways and on an unpredictable timetable as new social problems arise. The purpose of basic knowledge is to have some information "on the shelves" to retrieve as needed to address newly emerging social issues. Applied developmental science recognizes that social problems change faster than does our ability to generate useful information. As a result, it is essential to have research-based knowledge available that can be used to deal with new social problems or to guide research directly focused on those problems (Lerner, et al., 1994; McCall, 1996; Prewitt, 1980). By so doing, applied developmental science has the potential to rebuild collaborations between philanthropy and research.

The use of research on self-efficacy and self-esteem is one example. Research on these personal attributes provides important weapons to promote behavior changes aimed at reducing risk for HIV infection (Bandura, 1992). Yet no one expected that this research tradition would prove useful in this way because AIDS was not an epidemic at the time the research developed. On the other hand, research on a variety of existing youth problems (e.g., early adolescent sexuality and pregnancy, substance abuse prevention, reducing school dropout) has produced important information on adolescent development as well as addressing the particular problems of young people (Feldman & Elliott, 1990). Research is learning and learning needs to be part of social action, just as action should be triggered by the learning process.

Evaluations of social programs and interventions are one explicit form of directly "applied" research. Early efforts in particular emphasized a "black box" approach stemming from the social experimentation paradigm prevalent then. To some extent, this paradigm persists, and parallels a drug testing model. Individuals are randomly assigned to groups. Then one group receives an intervention, and selected outcomes are measured in the two groups. If there is a statistically significant group difference, it is safe to attribute causality to the one difference between the groups—the intervention. The standard experimental paradigm applies.

The problem is that interventions are not drugs. They are more complex in multivariate ways, and many factors other than the intervention affects the group outcomes. It is also not clear that random assignment can serve to obtain comparable groups in the contexts in which most social interventions are launched; and, often, random assignment is simply not possible in certain interventions (Hollister & Hill, 1995). In these cases, it may be more informative to ask what percentage of the variation in selected outcomes is accounted for by selected variables of the intervention. Most of what we know about youth development is based on quasi-experimental, correlational, or descriptive analyses. Children are not, for example, randomly assigned to good and bad parents; yet we attribute considerable importance to these non-experimental analyses of what constitutes effective parenting practices for children. Similar analytical strategies may prove useful in examining which variables of program participation relate to which participant's outcomes, and to what extent.

At the same time, many interventions are not set up as experiments and are not set up to accomplish much learning. They are established to heal, to help, and to promote the well-being of their recipients. Recent philanthropic efforts offer numerous examples. Yet all such interventions are based on models of change. The intervention is designed to include certain components thought to affect certain outcomes in the form of youth development or community change. In these cases, it is important to identify these implicit theories of change, because the intervention and research on it then becomes a test of that "theory of change" (Connell, Aber & Walker, 1995; Lerner, et al., 1994). That is, the evaluation then becomes theory-based research, contributing to knowledge about the phenomena addressed by the intervention as well as offering information on the effectiveness of a particular social program or policy. A logical extension of this position is to view interventions for youth as natural contexts for studying development and as important opportunities to contribute to our basic knowledge about developmental process (Sherrod, 1995, 1997b).

Applied developmental science is a perfect vehicle for promoting a new outlook on evaluation that both recognizes the potential for learning in all social change efforts and, at the same time, offers an array of tools other than the standard experimental paradigm for learning about the role of the intervention in the lives of the recipients. Indeed, from this view of evaluation, it also becomes a second-order intervention in that it empowers participants to take charge and restructure as they learn what is working, discover what is new, and generate new ways of solving old problems.

Philanthropy has important lessons to share in this regard, and university-based research has valuable expertise to aid philanthropy in promoting social welfare. In this regard, collaborations between universities, national independent foundations, and locally-based community foundations could be particularly effective. Science, however, offers an objectivity that is not inherent in this more grounded knowledge, which is vulnerable to, at least to accusations of, ideological bias.

Perhaps the most important achievement of applied developmental science is its recognition that communication between the policy or service or philanthropic communities and researchers should be bidirectional. That is, science has information to share with the policy and service communities. However, those individuals who serve children and youth in direct service as well as in public service or who use philanthropy to improve the public well-being also have questions to ask and lessons to share with the scientific community. That is, they too are an expert system (Lerner, et al., 1994; McCall, 1996).

In summary, applied developmental science can tap into private sources of funding by developing or renewing relationships with philanthropy of its various types. It can do so by bringing current research knowledge and methods to efforts at social improvement and can use the knowledge inherent in communities and in philanthropy to contribute to research agendas. It can preserve basic research in expectation of future needs as new social problems arise, and it can structure current efforts at social change by philanthropy (as well as by government and others) to insure that they contribute to our learning. Sherrod (1997a) also discusses these issues.

DISSEMINATION OF RESEARCH

Dissemination is a particularly critical ingredient of efforts to reconnect philanthropy and research. Research on child development provides much critically useful information of relevance to parenting and family decision-making and to the design and evaluation of programs and policies serving children and families. Yet, such information is too frequently relegated to academic journals and is not disseminated to the public, to the staff of programs serving children, to evaluators of such programs, to policy makers, or to funders and others who work on children's behalf. Such dissemination not only has the potential to improve the work that is done on children's behalf, but also is critical to maintaining a firm and substantial national commitment to funding research on child development.

Researchers are concerned with the quality of information. The purpose of researchers and research organizations in pursuing dissemination is to make information available to the full array of constituencies, public and private, that are concerned with the well-being of children and to policy makers and funders who set priorities and funding levels for scientific research. Because researchers' dissemination efforts do not proceed from a particular special interest, and do not advocate for particular purposes or positions, they maintain a political neutrality that does not always characterize other dissemination efforts. For this reason, dissemination or "giving child development knowledge away" as described by Richard Weinberg, former Chair of the Society for Research in Child Development's (SRCD) Social Policy Committee, is a particularly useful service for the research community.

The scientific community must take some responsibility for disseminating its findings to the public and to policy makers, for demonstrating the relevance of its work, and even for using that work to improve the general social good, as the early philanthropists wanted to do. For students of human development science-based dissemination is especially important, because it increases the chances that developmental issues are considered when policies are made for children, youth, and families.

Too often policies are determined not by individuals' developmental needs but by political considerations, together with social and institutional needs. The growth of mass public schooling in the U.S. is one historical example where social-economic rather than developmental considerations have disproportionately driven the formation of a major social institution for children. The Carnegie Foundation Report, *Turning Points* (1989), describes the problems that the growth of one component of public education, the middle schools, has created for young adolescents. The separation of middle schools, devoted to Grades 6 through 8, from elementary and high schools requires that children move to a new school and experience a sometimes bewildering variety of changes in peer groups and academic routine at a time that they are also experiencing the equally confusing changes of puberty. That is, the characteristics of this school structure in the U.S. conflict with the developmental needs of this age period; the growth of schools has been driven by factors such as overall population growth and the needs of labor rather than by the developmental needs of children and youth.

Private funders such as Grant, Carnegie, and MacArthur attempt to represent young people in bringing developmental issues to the public agendas for children and youth; the *Turning Points* report provides one such example. Applied developmental science offers an important opportunity for the scientific community to increase its role by joining with philanthropy in such dissemination efforts.

Broad-based dissemination, however, especially through the various media, requires both specific expertise and a network of relevant contacts. There are several points to be made based on this experience. First, even in a time of heightened legislative activity such as the present, the media are primarily interested in research information that is new and "ground-breaking" in some way. Relevance of known facts to policy decisions and implications of what we know for legislative directions are not sufficient to engage the media's attention. This indicates the need to educate the media, the public, and legislators about the general importance of research-based information. Information may not be the only factor influencing legislation as well as the public will, but it should make a contribution. This also indicates the need to help non-scientists understand the nature of research and to increase their interest in basic research as well as research immediately relevant to policies.

Second, locating relevant researchers who can serve as spokespersons to the media in specific, specialized fields is challenging and time-consuming. Yet the media are interested in such personal contact with the relevant researchers and local media are particularly interested in local researchers' perspectives. It is necessary to develop resource networks of researchers across the country who are ready and capable of communicating with the media and with legislators. And several of the current media specialists provide researchers with training in interacting with the various forms of the media. SRCD member Robert McCall has also written about this need, including a chapter in the Committee-produced *Handbook on Legislative Testimony* (1994).

Third, the developmental research community, at least a critical core of it, is interested in being mobilized to attend to dissemination, and some members are able to assemble in a clear, communicable fashion what is known in specific areas. Thus, it is feasible to develop a network of such researchers and dissemination is a reasonable and useful undertaking for the research community. But it requires sustained efforts and must rely on expertise in several areas.

There is, in fact, considerable nationwide interest in dissemination that can be mined. SRCD's Social Policy Committee has, in fact, prepared a directory of organizations across the country that are concerned with the dissemination of scientific knowledge to non-scientific audiences. This directory has already been circulated to the directors of these organizations as well as to select private foundations concerned with children. The directory represents the first systematic effort to establish some contact with the numerous national and regional efforts across the country oriented toward giving child development knowledge away. Approximately 80 centers and other organizations are included. Not all organizations are devoted exclusively to child development research, but all include some attention to the field. An update of this directory is needed and is currently underway.

Private foundations are particularly interested in dissemination, even more than in research itself. Dissemination, therefore, provides another important lever for initiating contact with philanthropy. Dissemination is, nonetheless, a difficult undertaking, and we need more research on dissemination itself. For example, what works, for what audiences, under what conditions? Also, how can we contribute to setting the agenda for what is covered by the media? A recent paper by Bonk and Wiley (1994) lays out numerous key issues and summarizes some lessons that have already been learned.

TRAINING

Funding of training will be the most challenging to encourage. It will be necessary to identify unusual avenues for training and coordinate efforts across these. There are already several discrete training programs across the country, for one year or a summer, aimed at providing policy-relevant experience for researchers. These are oriented to supplementing general graduate training in research. Because they are of limited scope, these programs are more fundable than general graduate training and, hence, should be expanded and further developed.

Applied developmental science, however, does increase the chances of private funding for training, for the same reasons that it increases the likelihood of support for research. The paper by Susman-Stillman and Brown (1997) describes some of the training opportunities across the country and summarizes training needs in applied developmental science from these graduate students' perspectives.

IN SUMMARY

Applied developmental science provides a vehicle for increasing private philanthropy's involvement with and funding for research. Its focus on university-community collaborations, dissemination of research, and training in applied research provides important opportunities for capturing the interest of philanthropy. Neither the field nor philanthropy can afford to miss these opportunities for partnership.

NOTE

Portions of this chapter are adapted from Sherrod, L. S. (1998). The common pursuits of modern philanthropy and the proposed outreach university: Enhancing research and education. In R. M. Lerner & L. A. K. Simon (Eds.), *University-community collaborations for the twenty-first century: Outreach scholarship for youth and families* (pp. 397-417). New York: Garland.

REFERENCES

Bandura, A. (1992). A social cognitive approach to the exercise of control over AIDS infection. In R. J. Diclemente (Ed.), *Adolescents and AIDS: A Generation in Jeopardy*. Newbury Park, CA: Sage Publications.

Bonk, K. & Wiley, M. (1994). *Communications strategies for policy agenda setting*. New Haven, CT: Quality 2000.

Cahan, E. D. (1986). *William T. Grant Foundation: The first fifty years, 1936-1986*. New York: William T. Grant Foundation.

Carnegie Council on Adolescent Development. (1989). *Turning points: Preparing American youth for the 21st Century*. New York: Carnegie Corporation of New York.

Connell, J., Aber, L. & Walker, G. (1995). How do urban communities affect youth? Using social science research to inform the design and evaluation of comprehensive community initiatives. In J. Connell, A. Kubisch, L. Schorr and C. Weiss (Eds.), *New approaches to evaluating community initiatives: Concepts, methods, and contexts*. Washington, DC: The Aspen Institute.

Feldman, S. S. & Elliott, G. R. (1990). *At the threshold: The developing adolescent*. Cambridge, MA: Harvard University Press.

Hall, P. D. (1988). Private philanthropy and public policy: A historical appraisal. In R. Payton, M. Novak, B. O'Connell and P. Hall (Eds.), *Philanthropy four views*. New Brunswick, NJ: Transaction Books.

Heimann, F. (Ed.). (1973). *The future of foundations*. Englewood Cliffs, NJ: Prentice-Hall, Inc.

Hollister, R. & Hill, J. (1995). Problems in the evaluation of community-wide initiatives. In J. Connell, A. Kubisch, L. Schorr and C. Weiss (Eds.), *New approaches to evaluating community initiatives: Concepts, methods, and contexts*. Washington, DC: The Aspen Institute.

Katz, B. & Katz, S. (1981). The American private philanthropic foundation and the public sphere, 1890-1930. *Minerva, 19*, 236-269.

Lerner, R. M., Miller, J. R., Knott, J. H., Corey, K. E., Bynum, T. S., Hoopfer, L. C., McKinney, M. H., Abrams, L. A., Hula, R. C. & Terry, P. A. (1994). Integrating scholarship and outreach in human development research, policy, and service: A developmental contextual perspective. In D. L. Featherman, R. M. Lerner and M. Perlmutter (Eds.), *Life-span development and behavior*. Hillsdale, NJ: L. Erlbaum Associates.

McCall, R. (1996). The concept and practice of education, research, and public service in university psychology departments. *American Psychologist, 51*(4), 370-388.

McCall, R. (1993). A guide to communicating through the media. In K. McCartney and D. Phillips (Eds.), *An insider's guide to providing expert testimony before Congress*. The Society for Research in Child Development.

Nason, J. (1989). *Foundation trusteeship: Service in the public interest*. New York, NY: The Foundation Center.

Prewitt, K. (1995). *Social sciences and private philanthropy: The quest for social relevance*. Essays on Philanthropy, No 15. Series on foundations and their role in American life. Indiana University Center on Philanthropy.

Prewitt, K. (1980). The council and the usefulness of the social sciences. *Annual Report of the President, 1979-80*. New York, NY: Social Science Research Council.

Renz, L. & Lawrence, S. (1993). *Foundation giving: Yearbook of facts and figures on private, corporate and community foundations*. New York: The Foundation Center.

Rosenberg, S. & Sherrod, L. (1994). *Directory of organizations concerned with public information of relevance to children*. Committee on Child Development, Public Information, and Public Policy. The Society for Research in Child Development.

Sherrod, L. (1997a). The common pursuits of modern philanthropy and the outreach university: Enhancing research and education. In R. M. Lerner and L. A. Simon (Eds.), *University-community collaborations for the twenty-first century: Outreach scholarship for youth and families* (pp. 397-417). New York: Garland.

Sherrod, L. (1997b). Promoting youth development through research-based policies. *Applied Developmental Science, 1*(1), 17-27.

Sherrod, L. (1995, June). Policy options for investing in youth. In *Invest in youth: Build the future, American Association of Family and Consumer Sciences research and policy agenda conference* (pp. 106-117). Alexandria, VA: American Association of Family and Consumer Sciences.

Susman-Stillman, A. & Brown, J. (1997). Building research and policy connections: Training and career options for developmental scientists. *Social Policy Report*, Newsletter of Society for Research in Child Development. SRCD: University of Chicago Press.

Universities in the Community: The Role of Trusts and Foundations as Facilitators for Social Change

Ulrike Schuermann
The Australian Youth Foundation, Inc.

On the eve of the twenty-first century, with information and technology substantially affecting traditional systems of learning and decision making, it is essential to scrutinize the relevance and effectiveness of our existing institutions, including universities. This entails analyzing the roles and functions of these institutions—in consultation with their "customers."

Unquestionably, universities are still central to knowledge production, innovation and distribution, and the contribution of scholars is of paramount importance to the further development of societies. Universities will still play an important role in producing the intellectuals, researchers and practitioners of and for the twenty-first century. They therefore have a responsibility to be progressive and pro-active—perhaps more so than other institutions. Universities also form an integral part of the community and as such must demonstrate leadership not only in regard to their core "business," but also and equally importantly, as socially responsible "citizens." Universities should work with communities in collaborative ways and orient their faculties and students to such efforts.

Issues such as globalization, unemployment, economic sustainability, the relevance of traditional education systems, and juvenile justice reform are posing complex challenges around the world—demanding more innovative and eclectic application of our collective intelligence. In a world struggling with seemingly insurmountable problems we cannot afford to keep our leading thinkers in the so-called ivory tower.

However, the current "compartmentalized" nature of many universities does not have the capacity to respond quickly to the complex challenges of the "global village." Designing solutions for the twenty-first century in partnership with government, corporations, trusts and foundations, not-for-profits and the public at large will require a more flexible and integrated operational structure and administration. Challenged to become more efficient through general public sector trends such as competitive tendering, restructuring, increasing privatization, and the introduction of businesslike management methods, many universities have already responded.[1]

It is not suggested we should further restructure or "rationalize"—rather, we should revive and revitalize. The first step to revive universities is through the renewal of their relationship with the society.

ONE FOUNDATION'S PERSPECTIVE

The reasons for university and community partnerships[2] are compelling, and the possible nature of the collaboration between universities and the community in the new millennium gives rise to this important discussion. Many universities and trusts and foundations share certain values and principles as a result of their idealistic and not-for-profit orientation.[3] The experience of the Australian Youth Foundation (AYF) might therefore be directly relevant to potential community-university collaborations.

This chapter presents one international perspective on this issue—based on the experience of the AYF. It is not an analysis of the university system[4] and its place in Australian society. Rather it shares anecdotal observations, made from one grant-maker's perspective in the hope that these will stimulate debate.

The AYF's mission is to assist socially, financially, physically or intellectually disadvantaged young Australians to reach their full potential. The strategies and programs adopted and implemented to achieve these aims and our experiences as a result provide the context for the view that trusts and foundations could facilitate interaction between universities and the community—to the mutual benefit of all parties.

In pursuit of its mission, the AYF has, since its establishment in 1988, funded more than 300 projects across Australia. The scope and activities range from public policy and program development to provision of technical assistance and the establishment of national advocacy bodies. The AYF has adopted a pro-active grant-making strategy and does not provide funds to unsolicited submissions, unless projects directly meet a priority area. Partnerships with other trusts and foundations, not-for-profits, corporations, federal, state and local governments, and the public at large have been actively developed and have greatly contributed to the reach and impact of the AYF's work and project partners.

Achieving long-term systemic change with and for children and young people is an integral part of our vision.[5] A comprehensive publications and communication strategy, as well as evaluation strategy, has been adopted to share our ideas, findings, and experiences with government policy makers and other relevant actors. Much effort and emphasis has been and continues to be placed on documenting innovative programs to replace anecdotal evidence with facts and thereby enhance the chances of influencing public policy. Furthermore, communicating our knowledge to educate key stakeholders, generating positive success stories about children and young people, and raising awareness of children's and youth issues in the community at large are seen to be among the AYF's primary responsibilities. All strategies adopted by the AYF draw not only on the expertise of children and young people, our board members and staff but also on independent advice from a variety of consultants, including leading academics and experienced practitioners.

RELATIONSHIP ISSUES

Partnerships with universities—essential to achieving the AYF's goals—have not always been easy or productive:

1. The AYF has initiated and funded action research projects involving individual academics as well as establishing public policy centers in partnership with universities, with additional resources made available for community consultations and demonstration projects. The purpose of funding public policy in combination with demonstration projects has been to provide new evidence of what works and to link research and practice. This provided the biggest challenge (in addition to the administrative issues described below) but it also created the greatest opportunity for universities to collaborate with communities.

2. The AYF has worked at different levels with the intellectual community, for example in the area of homelessness, juvenile justice and mental illness and has, in practice, explored a variety of ways of effectively engaging our intellectual community in social policy debate. Through its strategies of engaging both universities and community stakeholders, the AYF has been able to significantly influence the public policy debate on issues of growing importance and concern in North America, Europe and indeed in all regions. These include homelessness and the post de-institutionalization policy for the mentally ill, and are areas where we all have a great deal to learn.

3. A major impediment to the success of some university-based projects was the lack of flexibility and responsiveness of the university bureaucracy and its compartmentalization of responsibilities, particularly in terms of financial accountability. Thus, generic accounting policies are being applied without due consideration of particular circumstances. For example, at times universities have requested administration surcharges resulting in a grant of $50,000 costing $90,000 with the $40,000 added being only for administration of the grant. This is clearly very inappropriate in our specific case and short-sighted in terms of the long-term relationship with the community, particularly considering the opportunity provided to the institution through access to stimulating and real life course work or consultancies for its staff and students.

Universities need to recognize their responsibilities to the community (which supports them) and the value of investing their resources as a matter of course. These and other difficulties in the financial administration of grants due to centralized accounting systems is not an isolated problem and poses great challenges to program management. As a result, the success of projects is often dependent upon the motivation and ability of individuals or groups of academics to move around university bureaucracies.

4. Regardless of the nature of the programs, their success correlated directly with the readiness of the institutions and individuals involved to collaborate and focus on the common objective. The capacity to recognize each other's boundaries and compromise without compromising the values of the individuals or organization can either make or break a project. For example, the AYF funded one major university based project involving action research linked to demonstration projects managed by a joint committee. Conflicts caused by vested political interests and the belief that academic expertise and theory is more relevant than meeting the need of the community, combined with a total unwillingness to compromise, consumed valuable energy at the expense of constructive change.

Additionally, lengthy crisis meetings to negotiate a compromise with the highest level of authority were overturned by collective staff meetings. This imposed impossible negotiating circumstances, supported by the structure of the university. At the end of the funding period, it became evident that the university did not have a long-term commitment to the program.

BRIDGING THE GAP BETWEEN THEORY AND PRACTICE

The important issue of the relationship between theory and practice deserves further consideration. Trusts and foundations have unique experiences in working with all sectors of society and can act as facilitators aiming to bridge the gap between theory and practice. The experience in both research and service delivery places trusts and foundations in a unique position. Familiar with the strengths, weaknesses, and needs of both sides of the equation, trusts and foundations have the power through persuasion of prospective grants to facilitate communication and collaboration thereby fostering community and university partnerships.

Increasingly, universities are required to compete for corporate, public, and philanthropic funds with other not-for-profits. This has led to pressure on the institution to produce commercially tangible results and often caused a defensive attitude resulting in perceived "traditional" boundaries being protected at the expense of community collaboration programs that do not have a commercial orientation. Working collaboratively with the community is not conditional on giving up institutional independence or compromising the competitive edge. On the contrary, it may provide an opportunity to overcome these issues and add value to all facets of operations.

A common criticism of academics is the lack of practical relevance of course work. Complex theoretical concepts are best illustrated when applied to real life scenarios. Academics who have the opportunity to "test" theories throughout their career provide better and more relevant tuition. It is not suggested we abandon pure theory in favor of a purely practice-based attitude—but we have clearly reached a point when the quest for knowledge and innovation for its own sake is less important than an emphasis on effective application. It appears at times that some academics seek shelter behind theory to avoid the discomfort of reality and responsibility and that this behavior is accepted and supported within the structure of the institution. We need to create an environment that encourages application of theory, a certain amount of risk-taking and entrepreneurship combined with long-term commitment to achieving results. Of course, this also leads to responsibility and accountability and will demand a considerable amount of courage.

University-community collaborations offer opportunities for result-oriented research and learning in areas such as program development, evaluation, replication and assessment procedures, among others. They can therefore be instrumental in creating a new generation of applied researchers[6] to assist with the fundamental challenges confronting us.

CONCLUSIONS

The AYF has gained many insights about common strengths and weaknesses of programs and accumulated knowledge about what works and what doesn't, nationally as well as internationally. Having devised programs targeted at addressing multiple disadvantage (holistic) and impacting across disciplines (interdisciplinary) combined with technical assistance strategies, the AYF will now apply its expertise together with all local community stakeholders in addressing needs identified by local communities. A "community investment strategy" will be developed in order to impact specific geographic areas of high need including performance measures to assess impact throughout the process.

The contribution of and partnership with universities will be instrumental to the success of this "community collaboration" approach. The basic concept is one of community consultation aiming at bringing "best practice" programs to local practitioners. It is proposed, with the assistance of academics, to initially identify need, service delivery gaps and areas of duplication, then transfer knowledge and expertise where appropriate, and devise strategies incorporating performance measures for implementation of holistic programs addressing the needs of the community.

Universities should not simply view trusts and foundations as sources of funds to provide badly needed resources for research programs but as partners to find new ways to achieve positive long-term change.

The concept of full service schools,[7] which entails collaborative partnerships between schools and community agencies to address multiple needs of children and young people in the context of the family and the community, has become increasingly popular in Australia. Schools collaborate with families, health and mental health services, employment and housing services, police, local businesses and other relevant parties to address and redress the causes of social exclusion. Maybe the future concept for a relevant and appropriate university will be the "full service university," firmly based in the center of community activity and development.

In closing, it is precisely the increased accessibility and relevance of universities to their communities which could ensure their central role in the twenty-first century and also be one of the most important contributions to society at large. To achieve this, however, a more creative and inclusive approach in working with the corporate, public and philanthropic sectors is required.

NOTES

1.   Refer to "Civic Entrepreneurship" by Charles Leadbeater and Sue Goss, DEMOS and Public Management Foundation, UK, 1998.
2.   This relates in particular to the area of applied developmental science, e.g. psychology, sociology, social work in regard to training requirements, however, it is not restricted to these areas in regard to community involvement.
3.   Notwithstanding the pressure on most universities to be for-profit institutions.
4.   Australia's first university, Sydney University, was established in 1850 in Sydney; the number of universities has grown to approximately 42 universities today.
5.   The AYF's vision is that it will:

   •   Initiate constructive and progressive change; promote the integration and coordination of youth programs, services and policies; and establish its place as a respected and catalytic organization in youth affairs;
   •   Exhibit leadership in policy development, in the promotion of applied research, in fostering positive ideas for change and in acting as a facilitator for their implementation;
   •   Influence governments, academic institutions and the community; and
   •   Promote collaboration and networking in the youth sector.

6.   The AYF recently agreed to a work-placement arranged through the internet. A foreign social science student had to absolve several placements in community organizations as part of his course work over five years. He not only was an invaluable asset to the organization during his placement and added value through applying his knowledge to the AYF's work, but also he clarified his future professional career goals.
7.   The AYF funded the Australian Centre for Equity through Education—Better Schools for Better Future and provided funds to five different pilot full service schools sites. For further information about these programs please refer to the AYF web-site.

Afterword

Catherine J. Ross, *George Washington University*

In this book we have focused a great deal on scholarly engagement. I want to emphasize that scholarly engagement is not only altruistic. It is also self-rewarding and self-perpetuating. The cross fertilization involved when scholarship is engaged in the real world produces better and revitalized scholarship and that, in turn, revitalizes the work that we are doing in the community.

I think it also useful for each of us to remember why we chose our respective fields. I know many lawyers, particularly those who go into private practice, who went to law school for idealistic reasons. This background makes it easy to recruit them in efforts to serve children. I think that parallels to this example can be found in all of the fields represented in this volume. It is important for the students across the disciplines represented in this book to have as intellectual role models scholars like those contributing to this volume. The presence of such models allows students to know that—regardless of where their careers may lead them—they can return to scholarship that is both intellectually sound and valued by the academy and that such scholarship fits their idealistic goals of engaging in satisfying work that serves children and families.

The groups represented in this volume are a very powerful start in university-community coalition building. I use the word "start" because even though the contributions in this volume tell us that there is a lot of work that has already been done they indicate as well that we must work arduously to keep open the bridges that have been built and to capitalize upon them further. Simply, we have established important multidisciplinary conversations and new community-university partnerships; nevertheless, we are still learning about the principles involved in such work and about how to bring these efforts to scale in a sustained way.

It may be helpful to use the legal profession as a sample case of both what has been learned and about what may be understood in the future if we reach out across disciplines and professions to join universities and communities in efforts to promote better lives for children and families. I suggest that we begin to think about lawyers as potential allies. The legal profession is already doing a great deal to enhance the well-being of children merely through dealing with the law. For instance, the Steering Committee on the Unmet Legal Needs of Children of the American Bar Association (ABA) has, as a major part of its workload, been learning about what is being done for children by members of the legal profession and sharing this information so that colleagues are not reinventing the wheel. The Committee also works to identify needs that are not yet being met and then finds groups in the legal community that can meet them.

The members of the Committee think about such assistance in the broadest terms. People tend to think that lawyers think only about litigation and writing contracts. However, we are thinking also about children as our clients and encouraging the legal community to view them holistically, to think about them the way they think about corporate clients. As a result of such an orientation, lawyers are engaging in all kinds of youth-serving activities.

For example, the ABA recently published a book, *Make A Difference: 25
Projects for Lawyers*. This publication includes all sorts of activities, from
courthouse waiting rooms, to helping with adoptions, to helping families find
housing and healthcare. In addition, lawyers have set up daycare centers in housing
projects; they have then worked in these communities to help parents resolve other
issues where law can be useful.

As one example of the scope of this sort of effort, consider that state and local
bar associations are a very important part of this latter project. In order for both to
promote this work and to provide some minimum incentives and rewards, a
newsletter, the *Catalyst*, is produced. This publication presents the activities, not
only of all the ABA entities but also of state and local Bars and of law firms that are
doing good work for children. A recent issue of this publication presented a report
about a firm in Tallahassee, Holland and Knight, which is one of the leading firms
in Florida. This practice decided to consolidate all of its philanthropic efforts
through giving to a program called "Opening Doors for Children." The program is
open to all of the firm's staff, and involves bringing books to children centers,
reading one-on-one, and mentoring children and their families.

Similarly, the Family Law Section of the ABA held for the first time, in Spring
1997, a meeting in conjunction with the American Psychological Association.
Meeting in Los Angeles, participants talked about what they could learn from each
other.

Accordingly, as evidenced by the example of the legal profession, there are
many, many ways to fit one's discipline or profession into what is a national trend
for multidisciplinary and multi-professional integration with communities. Indeed,
echoing the views of James Votruba in this book, the timing could not be better.
The *Zeitgeist* is with us when we undertake such collaboration.

Using law once again as an example, we are seeing more and more law school
courses in the traditional case-law method and more clinical placements involving
children and families. Personally, I am part of a national effort to collect the child-
and family-relevant syllabi of all the courses being offered in law schools not only
to help the sharing of such information across institutions but also to give to law
students a tool to use as a negotiating point with their deans. The presence and
scope of, and the faculty involved in, the numerous instances of such courses allows
students, for instance, to appraise the top 20 law schools, note that all institutions
are offering courses, and are using tenured or tenure-track professors to teach them.
Having such information empowers students to argue for such courses at their
institution and/or to make the case that other than adjunct faculty should teach them.

Given the interest among members of the legal profession in children and in
programs supporting them, one should be in touch with the nearest Bar Association
and law school when working in local communities to build coalitions. Also, there
are law students who are eager to use their knowledge and skills for collaboration.
Indeed, this sort of collaboration was the highest priority of the Law Student
Association during 1997 and 1998.

Moreover, for several years such work has been and will continue to be the
highest priority of the young lawyers division of the ABA. Members of this division
are lawyers who are up to age 35 and who are still full of idealism and energy. Even
though they are building their practices, they find the time to do great work for
children and youth. They have opened children's waiting rooms in courthouses in
more than half of the states and there are plans for the rest of the states. There is a
Young Lawyers Division in every state and local Bar Association.

In reaching out to involve lawyers in coalitions, it is important to remain aware
that lawyers do not have the substantive knowledge of children and families that is
represented in the chapters in this volume and that is present among university
communities in general. The lawyers who want to devote their time to children need

the substantive knowledge that is possessed, then, by members of the American Association of Family and Consumer Sciences (AAFCS) and among the scholars involved in applied developmental science (ADS). In turn, the knowledge and skills of lawyers should be of use to scholars from these fields.

For instance, many academicians do not like to write testimony or give it. However, lawyers love to do this. Accordingly, if AAFCS or ADS scholars have data in need of presentation to policymaking bodies, lawyers can help to put it in the appropriate form and, typically, may be only too glad to stand before a microphone and present it. Lawyers can also help other scholars learn what is involved in preparing and presenting testimony to policy makers and how to get access to such people. Moreover, lawyers can call their clients. Many of these clients are leaders in the communities we wish to reach. Across this volume mention has been made of the utility of building bridges to businesses. Businesses are the clients of lawyers.

In sum, we all know the pressing issues facing America's youth. For instance, 100,000 children go to bed homeless every night in the U.S., and the devolution of services across the nation will have an as yet unknown impact on the quality of life of our nation's young people. Understandably, these issues create a sense of crisis and act as an impetus to get things done quickly. If immediate actions do not work, however, there is a risk that disappointment, frustration, and diminished motivation will result.

Across the chapters of this book there have been repeated calls for the transformation of universities and for the elimination of obstacles to such transformation. However, we do not know if eliminating obstacles is a realistic goal. I would like to suggest that there are two levels of goals: There is a *hortatory* level, which involves the long term. These are the obstacles that one should try to eliminate. In law, such obstacles are compared to those that exist on the *mandatory* level. At this level one may encounter obstacles (e.g., poor administrators in universities), but the goal should be to reduce, rectify, or some how get such obstacles under control.

We want to retain our vision of hortatory goals. We do not want to stop trying to change the world. But we also have to be realistic. It is a life's work to implement the numerous rich and varied ideas about university transformation and about building multidisciplinary and multi-professional collaborations with communities that are contained in this volume. This work will engage both the authors in this volume and, as well, their students and probably their students, in turn. Accordingly, our challenge is to retain our energy and passion for pursuing the multi-generational tasks that lie before us.

Two quotes suggest themselves as useful for framing the nature of this challenge. One is from a person who wondered why we have been so slow in America to follow modern devices used in other nations for minimizing dependency, "Why is it, that we are best at suggesting foster families rather than schemes for preserving the natural family of the father, the mother, and the children living as they were meant to live?" The speaker was Jane Addams, and the year was 1909.

I do not mean to suggest that the work done between 1909 and today was wasted. In fact, although we have work before us that will take generations to complete, we have come a long way. And here, then, the second quote, from Winston Churchill, is relevant: "This is not the end, it's not even the beginning of the end, but it is perhaps the end of the beginning."

Afterword

James C. Votruba, *Northern Kentucky University*

The power of a scholarly community is illustrated by the combination of ideas and actions that are presented across the chapters of this book. The vision for university transformation, for building bridges between university and community, that is present among the scholars who have come together in this volume reinforces for any single participant in such work the fact that one is not alone in pursuing the complex and often daunting work of university transformation. Understanding that one is part of the cutting-edge not only supports one's endeavors but also places one in a community from which further knowledge can be gained and within which co-learning can occur.

An article in a recent issue of *Change* magazine was entitled, "Researching for Democracy and Democratizing Research," (Ansley & Gavento, 1997). The article contained a very interesting passage: "The heart of the problem in linking research and democracy is not only the question of whose voices are strengthened by university research but, also, who participates in research in the first place," (p. 46). This article goes on to note that many communities long ago gave up on universities as places from which they could expect meaningful assistance. As an alternative, some communities have worked out ways to produce or simulate the knowledge that they needed from universities. The article provides a basis for arguing for the need to transform the role of university research in and with communities.

Beyond the value of this article *per se*, what is interesting to me is its very appearance in *Change*. Two years prior to its publication such an article would not have been likely to appear in the magazine. There was not a scholarly community visible enough to justify the use of limited journal space. However, now there is and the appearance of such an article both informs and reinforces this community.

Accordingly, the timing of the present volume could not be better. The vision and actions presented in this volume operationalize much of the significant work present across the nation in transforming universities in a manner that elicits and merits the public trust; this work defines centrally what we are or should be about as institutions of higher education.

The reason this nation has invested so lavishly over the last hundred years in higher education is not because it sees higher education as an end of itself; rather, this investment occurred because the nation and its policy makers saw higher education as linked to a broader social agenda. This association was seen when universities brought science to agriculture; it was true when universities educated the work force for industrial expansion; it was true during two World Wars; and it was true when we entered the era of universal access to education in the post-WW II period. Similarly, the use of higher education for furthering the broader national interest was seen in regard to national defense and the Cold War.

However, a key issue for higher education, one that we are just now beginning to understand, is the impact on universities of the ending of the Cold War. In the context of this new era we need to inquire into the extent to which these universities remain central to the life of our nation. It is my belief that scholars working on campus to help build and sustain connections with communities are forging a path that will be critical to the vitality of higher education in the twenty-first century, a period when Cold War-style national defense and issues of East-West competition (as opposed to collaboration within a global economic community) may not be as central as they may have been in prior historical periods.

Once again, then, the timeliness of the present volume is underscored. Our universities are being asked to be more publicly accountable, more "outcomes" driven, more connected with the public agenda, and more able to demonstrate value to a skeptical public. All of these demands make the transformational activities suggested in this volume, and the new scholarly community that is being created by virtue of the development of such work, requisite for inclusion in the mainstream of our universities.

Universities and their senior administrative officers are struggling to try to figure out what their world is going to look like in the twenty-first century. They are confronted by changing student demographics, changing public expectations, technology that allows for education to occur anytime and anywhere, globalization of higher education, new public/private alliances, and new funding formulae. The sand moves continuously in their world, for example, involving changes in federal research policy or changing demands of local legislators—who might press an institution at one time to make a difference in public schools and at another time to effect change in local economic development.

In the face of such changing pressures and unpredictability it is often the case that there is a vision vacuum on many of our campuses. Across the nation, senior administrative leaders are looking for new visions to sustain their institutions. I believe this situation represents an opportunity for the type of scholarship advocated in this book. Scholars of outreach, for example applied developmental scientists, can help contribute to that vision needed by provosts, presidents, and members of governing boards by demonstrating how such research, undergraduate and graduate training, and application represents both a viable approach to scholarship *and* a valued-added contribution by universities to communities. However, to add this component to the vision of senior administrative leaders we need to be able to fly at 30,000 feet and at tree-top height simultaneously. We need to be able to have a big picture of higher education in society and a view of what, within the frame of our own particular area of scholarship, needs to be accomplished with a specific community partner. Simply, we need to be strategic as well as visionary.

Catherine Ross's views of coalitions in this volume are an illustration of the dual orientation we need. She explains, for instance, how partnerships with national and local activities of members of the legal profession (e.g., with Bar associations) represent a strategy enabling our vision of university-community collaboration to be advanced. Her ideas suggest that there are many other partners in the community that may not be on our screen. However, we should broaden our screen and make sure we are incorporating as many different perspectives as possible.

Such coalition building and the new research, teaching, and application activities it will engender affirm the assertion of the new conception of scholarship that is embodied in this volume. This new view of scholarship makes it clear that new partners, both within and outside of the academy, need to be involved in scholarship. Such innovation will require the development of new standards for the evaluation of such scholarship. Work at Michigan State University is an example of such a development. The document, *Points and Distinction of Planning and Evaluation* (Sanamann, 1996), produced by Michigan State reflects this effort.

However, as illustrated by this publication, higher education must demonstrate that it is very good at assessing outcomes and impact. We have to be rigorous and frank with ourselves when our work may not hit the standards that we set for quality and quantity of productivity. Such standards require candor and intellectual honesty. We need to prepare faculty across the university to understand the nature of outreach scholarship—even if they will not be among those colleagues engaged in it. If we are to maintain academic freedom and the breadth and openness of the university community, we cannot anticipate (nor should we want) all colleagues to become outreach scholars. We need to be sympathetic to the point of view that runs counter to engagement in outreach scholarship. However, we need also to work at all of our institutions to insure that an equitable amount of funds are directed toward this kind of work and that colleagues who engage in it are evaluated fairly and rewarded appropriately.

But, again, we need to be strategic in promoting the acceptance of outreach scholarship within our university community. Here let me consider the role of provosts to illustrate why this is important. Provosts have a very high stack of problems on their desks. When they see somebody come through the door they are asking themselves, "Is this another problem or is this a solution?" Accordingly, in terms of a strategy for approaching provosts and other leaders on our campuses it may be better to position ourselves as individuals who are there to help alleviate some of the problems that are on the desks rather than as lobbyists on behalf of issues that will create other problems. For instance, as illustrated by several contributions in this volume, our work can be presented as a set of activities that supports undergraduate education. Involving undergraduates in outreach enhances the meaning and relevance of their education and adds value to the communities in which they work. For a provost, such a contribution by outreach scholarship to undergraduate education not only enhances the marketing of the university to potential students and parents but also, at the same time, makes connections with the general public. Such activities will help enhance public trust.

Simply, then, in making the case for outreach scholarship to our administrative officers, we would be wise not to cast our appeal primarily in terms of needing more money to accomplish our agenda. Rather, we should approach them in regard to how we are there to help them accomplish their agenda in new, important, and marketable manners.

Here, it is useful to recall Jack Levine's image of a lever to influence policy makers, whether they are in higher education institutions or in legislatures. We need to find ways to cast our knowledge in the ways that policy makers understand. Perhaps the major segment of the audience for this volume uses or at least understands the language of applied developmental science. But to leverage policy makers we need to find ways of expression that are accurate but not peculiar to our profession or discipline. Neither university administrators nor policy makers can make the case for our ideas if they use only the argot of our academic fields. For the public in particular such language is off-putting and a reason for the failure of the leverage we try to apply.

As I have noted, most university administrations are struggling to keep their heads above water. We need to arm them with a vocabulary about our efforts that will enable them to understand how what we do reduces their struggle. In addition, we need to go beyond words and bring them into a community and let them experience the full range of involvement that we have there. Armed with concepts that allow them to understand the scholarship we are pursuing, they should meet our community partners. They should listen to the community voices that can tell the story of the meaning of our work to them. I believe that such experiences will give university leaders, and perhaps especially members of governing boards new ways of feeling proud of their institution. Many board members do not get many opportunities outside of athletics to experience such pride and often they do not understand the academic intricacies of our work. Such community encounters will, in my experience, be events they can understand and appreciate.

Accordingly, university leaders should meet with community collaborators, not on campus, but in a public school or in a community non-profit organization. The staff and community people present can indicate how the world is a different place, or how their community is a better place, because of the work of the university.

In this way, we are capitalizing on Jack Levine's interesting point that, to use leverage effectively, we should be advocates not lobbyists. As illustrated by the idea of bringing university leaders to meet in the community with one's community partners, such advocacy is useful in ways both internal and external to the university.

The success of internal advocacy will be critical if the incentives and rewards for outreach scholarship, that I have noted need to be accepted on a institution-wide basis, are to become a reality. Here, however, such advocacy may need to occur on a unit-by-unit basis. It is very difficult in a university of forty thousand to try to change the reward system. But it is less difficult to identify units where outreach scholarship is consistent with a mission and where there may be some leadership to form a community to define a unit-based outreach mission that is consistent with the overall university mission, to provide definitions and criteria for evaluation, and to introduce measures of excellence.

We need to recognize that the scholarship of engagement has a different time line. For numerous reasons—involving career development and university reward systems—it is a lot easier to do this kind of work as a senior (tenured) faculty member than as a young assistant professor. As such, even in institutions where such scholarship is encouraged, young colleagues may do less of it. Such productivity makes it all the more important to evaluate quality and impact. There is a burden on senior colleagues in this appraisal. Senior colleagues versed in outreach scholarship need to interpret the quality and quantity of such work for colleagues who may not understand how much time it takes to do such scholarship and/or the standards of productivity that are appropriate.

Similar arguments may be made for teaching as well as for research. In fact, using teaching as an example of the new frames that will be needed in the academy for understanding the value of outreach scholarship will allow me to illustrate why members of the university community need to think outside of the traditional boxes when considering university-community collaborations. The way higher education institutions are organized for teaching is around undergraduate and graduate education. In fact, however, the fastest growing education market in this country is lifelong education. There are hundreds of thousands of people throughout the nation who are currently engaged in doing the work that undergraduate and graduate students are now just being prepared to do. But, the people currently engaged in this work need to continue their education. In addition, we have youth professionals all over this nation who are struggling to cope with youth development. They will get information and tools from somewhere to help them in their work and it seems to me they should be getting these resources from the university. Partnerships with community organizations, including Cooperative Extension, can provide access to and perhaps considerable support for such innovative teaching. Simply, to engage in such continuing professional education, we need to think about work across the life span and not just about graduate and undergraduate instruction.

Finally, I should note that in building the new communities of collaboration discussed in this book, it seems critical to recognize that passion, perseverance, and commitment are as important as the power of ideas. There is too little passion in universities today. There is too much concern about survival and too little focus on what we should be about in regard to teaching, research, and outreach. The contributions to this book indicate that there are powerful and unique ideas about university-community collaboration. I see as well a great deal of passion for accomplishing a lot. This critical linkage between powerful ideas and passionate action can be illustrated by a passage from a recent article (Schlender, 1998) from

Fortune magazine. In the article a CEO of a major corporation described a conversation that he had had with the management consultant, Peter Drucker. At the end of the conversation the CEO looked at Drucker and said that the conversation had been wonderful. Looking back at him, Drucker replied, "Don't tell me this has been a wonderful conversation, tell me what you're going to do different next Monday."

REFERENCES

Ansley, F. & Gavento, J. (1997). Researching the democracy and democratizing research. *Change*, *29*(1), 46.

Sanamann, L. (1996). *Points and distinction of planning and evaluation.* East Lansing, MI: Michigan State University.

Schlender, B. (1998). Peter Drucker takes the long view. *Fortune*, *38*(6), 162-173.

Appendix A
Curriculum

Denise Skinner[1], Heather Casto,
Thomas R. Chibucos, Virginia Clark, Mick Coleman,
Phyllis Davidson, Carolyn Drugge, Debra Gentry,
Mary Hager, Jan Hogan, Cynthia Johnson,
Julie Johnson, Margaret Kelly, Mary Ann Lewis,
Connie Ley, Ron Mullis, John Murray,
Frankie Denise Powell, Stephen A. Rollin, Ed Smith,
Mary Smith, Suzanna Smith,
Linda Vincent-Broussard,
Sue Whitaker, and Steve Wisensale

ACTION AGENDA

Develop general curriculum outline for courses in public policy engagement, which introduces the college student to the purpose, career opportunities, and theoretical and practical dimensions of public policy decision-making and evaluation.

RATIONALE

Support for family well-being must become a national priority. Research shows that when resources are available within the family and community, families can accomplish developmental transitions, complete tasks and functions effectively, and adaptively deal with the issues they face. The current status of children and families in the United States demands that we empower graduates to translate research into useful information for policymakers, enabling them to make informed policy decisions which contribute to the well-being of families.

As educators, our goal is to develop professional practitioners and active citizens who understand, participate in and give leadership to the well-being of families. While there are public policy courses in many institutions and various disciplines, they are, for the most part, designed by individual departments. They may only address existing policy as subject matter to be learned and understood. To develop individuals who can formulate, shape, evaluate and implement public policy initiatives, a different type of educational experience is required. There are a few institutions that address this concern in a collaborative and interdisciplinary manner. There are numerous ways courses might be implemented and there is a vast public policy arena. Nonetheless, such a process is developmental; pertinent understanding, knowledge and skills are best taught throughout the undergraduate and graduate experience with each new experience building upon previous learning and with recognition that each student will come to public policy engagement education with different levels of interest and experience.

To prepare the public policy strategist that are envisioned, the following goals, objectives and learning experiences are presented as aids to developing appropriate instructional modules, courses and experiences for infusion into a curriculum. Theses are representative and should not be viewed as all-inclusive. Instructors will need to establish objectives and learning experiences which are developmentally appropriate to the level and experience of students.

GOALS, OBJECTIVES AND LEARNING EXPERIENCES

Goals

4. Develop professional practitioners and active citizens who understand, participate in, and give leadership to policy formulation that supports individuals and families.
5. Provide a developmental process for student acquisition of public policy knowledge and skills through research, coursework, field experiences and mentoring experiences.

The following learning objectives and experiences provide a framework for accomplishing these policy education goals.

Learning Objectives

Students will:

1. Comprehend the types of political cultures and perspectives.
2. Identify sources of political and economic power and ways to use power as a resource in the policy process. Identify policy issues and stakeholders.
3. Analyze the multi-contexts and multi-perspectives of issues including demographic, economic, social, political, religious and historical, among others.
4. Engage in policymaking in all stages of the policy process including formation, implementation, evaluation, advocacy and education.
5. Forecast the effect of current policies on future needs as well as forecast future needs and issues.
6. Synthesize research for dissemination to diverse constituents.
7. Communicate knowledge about policy issues to appropriate policymakers, organizations and communities.
8. Describe the roles professionals play in the policymaking process.
9. Identify family issues at all stages of the life cycle.
10. Articulate multiple points of view related to family issues in an objective way.
11. Assess the impact of policy decisions upon the various contexts in which families live.
12. Build coalitions to address family issues.
13. Identify theories and models that guide policy formation and evaluation.
14. Understand policy impact analysis on different family forms, family members, and children of different socioeconomic and cultural backgrounds.
15. Understand ethical issues related to public policy formation.

16. Establish criteria for assessing policy, including developing explicit criteria from economic or social models, learning to justify criteria, and developing evaluation skills.
17. Understand the political process and power brokers, learning how to influence the process and how to build trust in relationships with leaders.
18. Learn how to build networks, coalitions and work groups.

Learning Experiences

Have undergraduate students:

1. Attend a public hearing, government meeting or political/advocacy group meeting and observe the policymaking process. Students will prepare a summary paper of their observations noting composition of the group (age, gender, ethnicity) decision-making styles used and who the key players are.
2. Select newspaper articles that report policy issues. Students will identify what the policy proposes, the underlying issues, for whom the policy is aimed, and the ideological values. Students will formulate their opinions of the positive and negative outcomes of the policy and the potential outcomes for families.
3. Select a cause, program, or pending legislation of interest to them and upon which government policies have some effect. Students will write a letter to the appropriate public official expressing their views and asking for support.
4. Prepare a research paper which focuses on a policy which affects families. Students will review the relevant research identifying the social, political and historical issues that have impacted on their topic. Then describe the policy and programs associated with it and their relevance to families. Use Ooms and Preister's (1988) Family Impact Analysis principles to conduct family impact analysis on the policy.
5. Study the resolution process and determine how it can be used to shape public policy. Students will write a resolution and plan how it could be moved forward to the point that it affects public policy.

Have graduate students:

1. Develop a research agenda that is pertinent to family policy.
2. Visit agencies and internship sites to understand better the scope of the policy network.
3. Utilize classroom simulation of a forum, engaging in debates around public policy questions.
4. Utilize case studies with simulated activities.
5. Identify theses and dissertation topics that focus on policy content and outcomes.
6. Utilize government reference section of literature.
7. Identify internships with agencies on policy evaluation.
8. Conduct family policy research or program evaluation research and disseminate findings to policy makers.
9. Write a white paper analyzing a specific issue that impacts families.

NOTE

1. For this appendix and the other ones in this volume, the lead author served as a group recorder at the Third National Conference on Applied Developmental Science which was held in March, 1997 and took responsibility for developing this set of recommendations. All other authors are listed in alphabetical order.

REFERENCE

Ooms, T. & Preister, S. (1988). *A strategy for strengthening families: Using family criteria in policymaking and program evaluation.* Washington, DC: The Family Impact Center.

Appendix B
Experiential Learning

Golden Jackson, Joyce Arditti, Ann Chadwick,
Alisa Ghazvini, Sue Jolly, Ethel Jones, Janet Kistner,
Charles McClintock, Cherlyn N. Nelson,
Catherine Solheim, Earline Strickland,
Jeanne Warning, Brian Wilcox, and Margaret Zusky

ACTION AGENDA

Set objectives for experiential learning opportunities in the public policy arena for undergraduate and graduate education.

RATIONALE

Effective public policy experiences offer exposure to the public policy process. Students observe and participate in various components of the policymaking process, including defining problems, collecting data to describe problems, developing and debating public solutions to problems, analyzing statements of conflicting and diverse political viewpoints, building coalitions and negotiating compromise. Students increase their understanding of the public policy process and its impact on individual and family well-being.

NEED

Building experiential learning opportunities in public policy begins with faculty commitment. Faculty involvement is essential to ensure continuity and trust between the university and community. Faculty support is needed for building a curriculum with experiential learning opportunities. Thus, the initial task in development of a public policy experience is faculty recruitment and development. Faculty committed to the importance of experiential learning are key to design of experiences that provide effective linkage between classroom knowledge, field application, and reflection. Conceptual development of experiential learning is followed by design of specific experiences.

OBJECTIVES AND STRATEGIES

Educational Objectives

   10. Develop understanding of connections between politics, policy, and service delivery.

11. Provide opportunities to interface with, understand, and appreciate a diverse, complex and changing world environment.
12. Instill value for advocacy and civic responsibility.
13. Provide opportunities for practice as data interpreter/translator.

Strategies

1. Determine the role of public policy experiences in the curriculum.
2. Examine current courses to identify opportunities for providing experiential learning.
3. Adapt existing courses.
4. Develop new courses (due to finite resources, some courses may be eliminated).
5. Identify community/policy agencies with content linkages appropriate for the unit.
6. Design content, timing and sequencing, monitoring/supervision, and evaluation of experiences.
7. Specify competencies to be achieved through experiential learning.
8. Design prerequisites for experiential learning:
   - What level and content of conceptual and professional development is necessary for effective participation, appropriate to level of experience?
   - What course work is necessary for basic literacy in the field, appropriate to level of experience?
   - What course work provides understanding of policy process, appropriate to level of experience?
   - What course work is necessary to provide adequate written, oral and visual communication skills?
   - What experiences/course work provide insight into cultural diversity and the ability to work effectively with and deliver services to individuals and families from diverse backgrounds?
9. Encourage a wide range of experience options, for example, research and policy development.
10. Offer a variety of experiences, ranging from one-time, in-class to full-term internships. Utilize more comprehensive, intense, detailed, and full-term experiences in upper division undergraduate or graduate courses.
11. Develop measures of competency achievement.
12. Develop collaborations with potential placement sites.
13. Collaborate with colleagues in other fields (e.g., social work) who have developed models or guidelines for experiential learning.

Appendix C
Changing University Culture
Julia Miller, Jean Bauer, Wendy Crook, Marguerita Furness, Gregory Hand, Shirley Hymon-Parker, Clara Pratt, Christine Readdick, Bea Smith, Retia Walker, Richard Weinberg, and Stephan Wilson

ACTION AGENDA

Cultivate, celebrate and rekindle a university culture that will foster university-community engagement.

RATIONALE AND GUIDING PRINCIPLES

As public universities attempt to maintain their historic relationship to the people they serve, there continues to be a disconnect between the values of academia and the role of universities in meeting pressing societal needs. In the past decade, public accountability for universities has brought increasing attention to the core values of the professoriate and many universities have been forced to re-examine policies regarding undergraduate education and promotion/tenure, among others. Yet, the need to strengthen university ties to communities is still a critical concern, especially because of perennial societal issues regarding children, youth and families and the role that universities can play in enhancing their lives. To increase university-community collaborations and to ensure their effectiveness, the culture within universities needs to be transformed. The following outlines objectives and strategies that can assist universities in developing the culture that will foster university-community engagement.

All engagement activities in the service of children, youth and families must be guided by and committed to principles of mutuality, reciprocity and capacity building. Objectives and strategies must reflect a strong appreciation for the complexity of systems change, the uniqueness of every university and the context of their diverse communities.

OBJECTIVES AND STRATEGIES

Objectives

14. Cultivate an environment that promotes and reinforces the capacity of the university to work with multiple communities to create a good society.
15. Increase the respect, resources and rewards for a range of scholarly investments in engagement.

Strategies

1. Encourage students, faculty and other constituents to be participants in community engagement through knowledge, values and advocacy.
   - Make use of university traditions, legacy and already established resources.
   - Provide incentives for the sharing of resources between and in the university and the community by increasing capacity of the university for community collaboration.

2. Identify and eliminate obstacles to collaboration, cooperation and partnerships.
   - Create communication networks which foster university-community engagement.
   - Establish organizational structures that promote collaborations.

3. Develop internal and external support for applied developmental science.
   - Build support for outreach scholarship into the university's strategic plan.
   - Acknowledge and give prestige to faculty, staff, students, and community members who build partnerships.
   - Identify and recognize central and other administrators who promote university-community collaborations.
   - Identify economic contributions of collaborations; for example, external funds generated, internal and in-kind resources, curriculum developed, and the value added to communities and the university.
   - Develop and identify outlets for peer review of applied scholarship.
   - Strengthen the rewards for university-community engagement and applied scholarship in the university.

Appendix D
Funding Opportunities

Norma Burgess, Nancy Bell, Ann Blackwell,
Lillie Beasley Glover, Gladys Hildreth, Jennifer Park,
Greg Sanders, Mary Ellen Saunders,
Lawrence Schiamberg, Lonnie Sherrod,
Robert Simerly, and Michael Smyer

ACTION AGENDA

Set objectives for funding policy-related activities in applied developmental science.

RATIONALE

Effectively linking philanthropy to community support and development is critical in addressing real world issues. Professionals in applied developmental science are positioned to listen to the needs of the community so that research may be guided toward practical application. Establishing relationships and partnerships within the community is essential for successful collaboration. Foundations, agencies and other funding sources are key in the implementation of collaborative activities.

OBJECTIVES AND STRATEGIES

Objectives

4. Effectively link philanthropy to community support and development to address issues.
5. Develop issue-based collaborations with communities and potential funders.
6. Develop multi-level initiatives appropriate for undergraduates, graduate, and lifelong education.
7. Develop new sources of funding for applied developmental science activities in priority areas.

Strategies

1. Articulate vision and mission of applied developmental science to key groups including communities and funders.
2. Emphasize the range of activities that could be undertaken by a multidisciplinary university-community collaboration.
3. Develop intra-university collaborations.

4. Collaborate with community knowledgeables to identify community priorities and university capacities.
5. Create models of collaborations with key stakeholders.
6. Establish and maintain relationships with potential funding sources.
7. Match community priorities with funding priorities of potential grantors.
8. Provide undergraduate and graduate students with opportunities to develop grantsmanship skills.
9. Initiate stronger policy focus in undergraduate, graduate, and life-long education.
10. Capitalize on changes in family foundations to provide endowments for activities.
11. Engage in Internet searches of funding sources at the local, county, state, federal, and corporate levels.
12. Encourage community leadership in solicitation of external funds.
13. Develop short- and long-term strategies that build on a cycle of refinement, success, dissemination, and program development.
14. Enhance grants activities and infrastructure.
15. Assure development and continuation of funding to sustain applied developmental science policy activities.

Name Index

Subject Index